To Dr
Health, happiness &
Peace

What Should I Eat?

Book 1– Discovering Your Ideal Diet

Rudy Scarfalloto, D.C.

© Copyright 2013, Rudy Scarfalloto

All Rights Reserved.

No part of this book may be reproduced, stored in a retrieval system, or transmitted by any means, electronic, mechanical, photocopying, recording, or otherwise used without written permission from the author.

ISBN-10: 1492758116
ISBN-13: 9781492758112

Serenity Press

Readers' Comments

"Dr. Rudy is ahead of his time. Finally a book that actually tells us how we can select our food with confidence! He takes the confusion out of the equation and leads us to an answer."
— Michelle Irwin, H.H.P, Raw Vegan Chef, Certified Lymphologist

"*What Should I Eat?* is inspiring. It supports readers in getting in touch with their own best consultant, their own body, their own intuition."
— Linda Westman, D.C.

"Dr. Scarfalloto's book is a must read if you are interested in food and health. In addition to guiding you in choosing the best diet for you, he provides a clear survey of the major diets, he gives insight into our ancestors' diets and discusses emotional eating, and tops it off by discussing the ethics of eating.
— Vivian V. Knispel, Ph.D. former humanities professor and Fulbright scholar.

"Have you ever wished that there was a convenient, clear, concise, thorough, and objective review of all the diets and eating plans that are promoted? Now there is! Dr. Scarfalloto's in-depth description of the historical, emotional, physical, social, and ethical considerations of how humans eat is engagingly presented, so each of us can thoughtfully consider what feels right for us. No pressures, no dogma, no heavy-handed pronouncements, or scare tactics...just the facts, offered with great love and respect! Thank you Dr. Rudy!"
— *Honey Judith Rubin, author of When the Smoke Clears—Who are YOU?...9 Steps for Becoming a Nonsmoker.*

"Another great book from Dr. Rudy Scarfalloto! I think he's got a real winner in this one. This book plows right through the confusion, and creates a clear path for the reader. I also like the way that he doesn't make judgments one way or the other about people's food choices. I especially like the idea of tuning in to your body's wisdom about what you should eat."
— Donna Overall, editor

"The quintessential question for anyone who is trying to eat healthy, lose weight or just feel better — "What should I eat?" In his book of the same title, Dr. Rudy Scarfalloto takes a lot of the mystery out of those four little words. By sharing his knowledge and passion for healthy living, in his own way filled with humor and insight, Dr. Rudy allows even the most lost individual to find their way to the proper diet for them and their journey to healthy living. I highly recommend this book to anyone who wants to go beyond the basics and delve into the heart of good eating and proper nutrition."

– Jeremy Taylor, LMT, CKTP, Anatomy and Physiology Instructor.

"Dr. Scarfalloto's book was a delight to read. It is very well written, and should be a "must read" for anyone who is trying to work through the web of information and misinformation on diets, whether for weight control, improving health, or maintaining health. He told me that one of his aims in writing this book was to provide unbiased information about the different types of diets. In this he has succeeded. His categorizing them in the manner that he does is no less than brilliant, allowing him to describe, in clear understandable terms, both the benefits and deficiencies of most of the major diets in vogue today. I fully agree with him that both variation and moderation are key factors in selecting and eating foods, and especially that diets must be individualized with the person having the ultimate responsibility for making that choice. There is no one diet that fits everyone's needs! My hat goes off to Rudy, and I thank him for letting me read it in advance of publication. I found it to be both useful and enlightening."

– Howard L. Silverman, Ph.D., D.C., board of directors for the American Academy of Functional Medicine.

OTHER BOOKS BY RUDY SCARFALLOTO

The Dance of Opposites
Cultivating Inner Harmony
The Edge of Time
Nutrition for Massage Therapists

Acknowledgements

My thanks to Jeremy Taylor, Honey Judith Rubin, Aubrey Lewis, Barbara Komlos, Vivian Knispel, Howard Silverman, Donna Overall, and Janet Young for their editorial assistance.

Special thanks to my brother, Joe, for filling in the details regarding food production in our hometown that I was too young to remember.

Table of Contents

Introduction ix

Part I: The Basics

Chapter 1:	Healthy eating in a Nutshell	3
Chapter 2:	The Language of Nutrition	7
Chapter 3:	The Nutrients	15
Chapter 4:	The Food Groups	33
Chapter 5:	The Other Side of Nutrition	49
Chapter 6:	Guidelines for Healthy Eating	61

Part II: The Diets

Chapter 7:	The Diets of Our Ancestors	69
Chapter 8:	How to Evaluate Any Diet	93
Chapter 9:	Survey of Major Diets	101
Chapter 10:	Okay, Let's Eat	137

Part III: The Bigger Picture

Chapter 11: Emotional Eating and Instinctual Eating	151
Chapter 12: How the Author Eats	163
Chapter 13: The Ethics of Eating	181
Chapter 14: Summary and Final Musings	209
Appendix A:	219
Appendix B:	221
Appendix C:	223
Appendix D:	225
End-notes and References	229
Index	245

Introduction

The title of this book asks a question to which I offer two possible answers:
- Eat what your instincts tell you to eat.
- Eat generous amounts of fresh fruits and vegetables.

Either strategy, properly applied, can lead you to your ideal diet. Furthermore, in my experience, the two work very nicely together. As I explain later in this book, the presence of fresh and unprocessed fruits and vegetables in the diet offers a number of benefits — one of which is easier access to our food instincts. Why? Quite simply, our food-radar is fundamentally designed for these foods, as explained in chapters 7 and 11. Likewise, as we gradually reawaken our natural eating instincts, we are likely to spontaneously favor more fruits and vegetables.

I am not suggesting here that you should eat fruits and vegetables to the exclusion of all other foods, or even that fruits and vegetables should form the bulk of your diet. The essential message of this book is as follows: *Unprocessed fruits and vegetables promote vibrant health, as well as allowing easier access to your instincts — which will then guide you to any other foods you might need, in the amounts appropriate for you.*

Yes, it really is that simple. However, "simple" is not the same as "easy." There are a number of complicating factors that prevent most of us civilized folks from eating in this very simple and, ultimately, natural manner.

In two of my other books, *The Dance of Opposites* and *Cultivating Inner Harmony*, I describe how to invite simplicity into your life. The secret is to allow simplicity to be in harmony with complexity. When the two are harmonious, complexity leads back to simplicity, as easily and naturally as the night ushers in the day. In the present case, the complexity of nutritional science fulfills its purpose when it guides us in discovering a simple diet that meets our needs.

One major factor that complicates food selection is the tangling of nutritional needs and emotional needs. This tends to "scramble" our access to our inborn food instincts, as discussed in chapter 11. Without easy access to our food instincts, healthy eating is difficult at best. Furthermore, our emotions are very much connected with our social and spiritual needs, which also powerfully influence our food choices, as described in the final two chapters of this book.

Rudy Scarfalloto, D.C.

    No matter how much we educate ourselves on nutrition, eating is likely to remain complicated and confusing until it is restored to the simple, pleasurable and instinctual act that it was designed to be. This book, like other nutrition books, is a journey through the complexity of nutrition and food selection. One of my goals has been to be thorough. My other goal has been to present this complex body of knowledge in a way that guides the reader to the simplicity of eating according to instincts, so meals are easy to prepare and enjoyable to eat, while promoting long-term health and longevity.

    May your journey through this book be a joyful one.

Part I
THE BASICS

Healthy Eating in a Nut Shell

The Language of Nutrition

The Nutrients

The Food Groups

The Other Side of Nutrition

Guidelines for Healthy Eating

Chapter I
Healthy Eating in a Nut Shell

This chapter is essentially a "digested" version of the core principles for healthy eating, explored in greater detail in the chapters that follow. This will give you the option of applying the principles right away, even though you may not yet have all the pertinent details for understanding the subtleties of nutrition.

Some teachers of nutrition, myself included, are of the opinion that healthy eating requires that we take into account individual differences. Others believe our differences are relatively minor, and, therefore, promote pretty much the same diet for everyone. However, there are some points on which virtually all teachers of nutrition agree, as described below.

The Nutrients

The bulk of the food on your plate typically consists of carbohydrates, fats and protein, with much smaller amounts of the various vitamins, minerals, and phytonutrients. Here are the functions of these nutrients:

- *Carbohydrates* are the preferred fuel of the body. Most of the carbohydrates you ingest are burned (broken down) to provide us with the energy we need to stay alive and healthy.
- *Fats* have several functions, such as providing us with an important second source of fuel, so the body is not totally dependent on carbohydrates. In addition to their fuel value, fats are used to build our tissues, especially the brain and nerves, as well as providing regulatory functions.
- *Protein* is the bricks and mortar of the body. In other words, protein is the major building material for making our bones, muscles, skin, nerves, blood vessels, and internal organs. Protein can also be burned for energy, but the body prefers to keep this to a minimum, because it results in the formation of toxic byproducts.

- *Vitamins and minerals* are used mainly for their regulatory roles. In other words, they are not burned as fuel or used as building material, but rather to regulate how the body works. For example, they regulate how the body burns fuel and builds tissues. Therefore, they are needed in smaller amounts compared to protein, carbohydrates, and fats.
- *Phytonutrients* are thousands of plant-derived chemicals that are used mainly for their regulatory roles.

Key Principles for Good Nutrition

Opinions vary regarding the requirements for above nutrients. Furthermore, in recent years, other dietary points have been made:. For example:

- **Get Adequate Amounts of Fiber.** We need an abundance of plant fiber to maintain a healthy digestive system.
- **Balance Cleansing Foods and Building Foods.** Building foods are the ones rich in proteins, carbohydrates and fats. Cleansing foods include most fruits and green leafy vegetables, especially in their raw state. Cleansing foods tend to be rich in fiber and water. Green leafy vegetables are also very rich in chlorophyll, the chemical that makes plants green. Chlorophyll is Mother Nature's own internal cleanser.
- **Get Adequate Amounts of Raw Foods.** Ideally, we should consume some food in its raw state because cooking, especially at higher temperatures, destroys many nutrients and generates byproducts that may be toxic to the body, including some potent carcinogenic (cancer causing) substances.
- **80% Alkaline-forming Foods and 20% Acid-forming Foods.** Alkaline-forming foods leave an alkaline residue in the blood, while acid-forming foods leave an acidic residue. In order for the body to be healthy, it must have the proper acid/alkaline balance. To achieve this, the diet should consist of 80% alkaline-forming foods and 20% acid-forming foods.

The main alkaline-forming foods are fruits and vegetables. Acid-forming foods include animal products and most grains, nuts, and seeds. The typical diet in industrialized nations, consisting mostly of acid-forming foods, increases the toxic burden on the body and promotes degenerative diseases, such as osteoporosis, and accelerates aging. Likewise, a favorable acid/alkaline balance encourages cleansing and regeneration, lessens painful conditions, and promotes mental clarity and emotional calmness.

- **Avoid Excessive Animal Products.** Excessive amounts of animal products can overburden the body with toxic residue and produce deficiencies. The toxicity can occur on several levels, such as over-acidifying the body, and causing the accumulation of excessive iron. The deficiencies are due to the lack of numerous vitamins and minerals, and total absence of phytonutrients, found in fruits and vegetables. In other words, even if the animal products do not become toxic in large amounts, their unrestricted consumption effectively "pushes out" the fruits and vegetables, thus creating deficiencies.

  The combination of toxicity and deficiencies contribute to the onset of degenerative diseases, such as heart disease, cancer, and arthritis. Therefore, individuals who eat animal products should be mindful of not just "filling up" on these foods, but rather to leave room for generous helpings of cleansing foods.

  Regarding the appropriate amount of animal products, I hesitate to suggest a specific quantity that can apply to everyone. This is where I would advise you to educate yourself about your personal needs. However, the 80/20 principle described above seems to provide a good reference point to begin the process of discovering your own personal needs.

- **Avoid Excessive Grains.** The reasons for being conservative with grains are similar to those that call for moderation with animal products. In other words, unrestricted grains can produce toxicity and deficiencies. For example, grains tend to be acid-forming, though not as much as animal products. Grains also tend to be lower in vitamins and minerals and phytonutrients than fruits and vegetables, and can, therefore, lead to deficiencies — especially if the bran has been removed, as is often the case. In addition, grains contain phytate, which may pull minerals out of the body. Many grains also contain gluten and other proteins that can trigger allergic reactions in many individuals. The grain that tends to be the most problematical is wheat, because the modern strains have been heavily hybridized. Therefore, as with animal products, do not just fill up on grains, but rather eat them in amounts that allow you to feel satisfied, while still leaving room for the cleansing foods.

The above information might seem a bit much to juggle, but the good news is that all of these concerns tend to be automatically addressed by simply using the following rule of thumb: *eat an abundance of high-water content foods.*

High-water-content foods are the ones that produce copious amounts of watery juice when put through a juicer. These foods include most fruits and vegetables, as well as the young tender sprouts and shoots of grains and legumes. Here are some benefits of eating an abundance of high-water-content foods:
- We tend to automatically eat the right amount of protein, carbohydrates, and fats.
- We tend to get an abundance of vitamins and minerals.
- We get an abundance of plant fiber.
- We establish a good balance of cleansing foods and building foods.
- We establish the right balance of acid and alkaline forming foods.
- We reduce the consumption of processed foods in the diet.

How do you know if you are consuming the right amount of high-water-content food? In general, if you consume enough of these foods to have 1-3 bowel movements per day (which do not smell too bad), you are probably in the right ballpark.

Bless Your Food

There is more to good nutrition than chemistry and physiology. Whether we are aware of it or not, food is, for most of us, a highly charged emotional issue. After mother's touch, food is the first form of comfort we receive outside the womb. Even for adults, food is a major source of pleasure and comfort, as well as being a vehicle for social interaction. In addition, many cultures attach spiritual or religious significance to food.

Regarding the effect on the body, our emotional state has a great impact on how the body processes food. In particular, our attitude toward the food itself can influence the body's ability to handle it. The more we appreciate and enjoy the food, the more thoroughly we tend to digest it.

Chapter 11 examines this topic closely, because the emotional side of eating is often the factor determining whether or not a given diet "works" for a given individual. For now, the bottom line is this: after you have made your food choice, bless it, give thanks, and enjoy.

Chapter 2
The Language of Nutrition

What is a nutrient? What is a toxin? What is medicine? What is a sugar? What is a complex carbohydrate? What is metabolism? Popular authors often bend the definitions of these terms — the same word can be used in different ways by different authors. Such a lack of consistency tends to confuse an already complex subject. Therefore, let us begin by providing clear definitions for the common terms used in the study of nutrition.

Food and Nutrients

Food is the stuff we eat. Nutrients are the chemicals that our bodies extract from food, so as to maintain life. Once we grasp the distinction between food and nutrients, we would not say, "Wheat is a carbohydrate." We would understand that wheat is a food, while a carbohydrate is just one of the nutrients found in wheat. We would therefore correctly say that wheat is rich in carbohydrates, while also understanding that wheat contains other nutrients, such as protein, fats, and a variety of vitamins and minerals. Similarly, we would not say, "Salmon is a protein." Instead, we would say that salmon is a rich source of protein, while providing other nutrients as well.

To illustrate how lack of consistency with terminology might contribute to confusion, take the example of beans. In the past, I have heard some individuals say, "Beans are a protein." Others would come back with, "No, beans are a carbohydrate." In reality, beans are neither a protein nor a carbohydrate. Beans are a *food* containing protein, carbohydrates, and a bunch of other nutrients. From that perspective, we would understand that beans are, indeed, a significant source of protein, but they also contain a much higher level of carbohydrates.

Whole Food

By understanding the distinction between food and nutrients, we can fully appreciate the concept of *whole food*, which is any food containing all the nutrients naturally found in it. For example, an orange is a whole food. On the other hand, cheese is not a whole food; it is an extract consisting mostly of protein and fat. In other words, cheese has an unnaturally high concentration of some nutrients, which means that it also has to be deficient in others. This is significant, because the high concentration of protein and fat could overburden the digestive system, while the lack of other nutrients will essentially "rob" the body of these nutrients. The same applies to any food-extract, such as vegetable oil, butter, or tofu.

An important concept for good nutrition is to favor whole foods, while avoiding or exercising moderation with any food having a nutritional profile that has been altered from its natural state. From this perspective, we can understand why some authors argue that the term "whole food" should only be used for raw and relatively unprocessed foods, because heating and other forms of processing can destroy many nutrients. However, most authors would disagree with this idea or simply ignore it, since it would exclude foods forming the basis of most diets.

Furthermore, to select whole food that is really wholesome, we should bear in mind that any food will have other chemicals in it besides nutrients, as shown in figure 2.1.

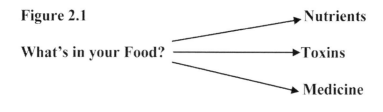

Figure 2.1

What's in your Food? → Nutrients / Toxins / Medicine

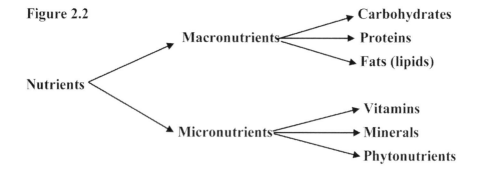

Figure 2.2

Nutrients → Macronutrients → Carbohydrates / Proteins / Fats (lipids)

Nutrients → Micronutrients → Vitamins / Minerals / Phytonutrients

The nutrients get virtually all the attention, while we tend to ignore the other factors. Even when we do address them, we freely use the terms, "nutrients," "toxins," and "medicine," but usually do not have a clear definition for each one. By gaining such understanding, we can better nourish ourselves, use medicine more wisely, and avoid poisoning the body.

We can begin to understand the distinction between the three by first taking a closer look at nutrients. For convenience, nutrients may be placed into two categories: macronutrients and micronutrients, as shown in figure 2.2.

Macronutrients form the bulk of the food on your plate (macro = large). In contrast, micronutrients are needed in relatively small amounts. Now the question is, how does the body use nutrients? How do we describe their "nutritive" function?

The Body Uses Nutrients in Three Ways

The distinction between nutrient, toxin, and medicine becomes clear when we recognize the three fundamental ways in which the body uses nutrients:
- They are burned as fuel
- They are used as building material
- They provide regulatory functions

Nutrients as Fuel

Nutrients serving as fuel are simply broken down or "burned" for energy, which is measured as calories. Since the body needs a lot of energy, nutrients burned as fuel must be ingested in relatively large amounts.

Nutrients as Building Material

While fuel is burned for energy, building material is assembled like bricks and mortar to form our flesh and bones. Nutrients used as building material are needed in lesser quantities than nutrients burned as fuel. This is easy to understand when we remember that fuel has to be continually replaced in large amounts, while building material must be replaced only to allow for growth, repair, and maintenance. As an analogy, wood can be used to build and repair your house, as well as to heat your house. Ultimately, you need more wood to heat your house than to build and repair it.

Naturally, a growing body needs more building material than one that is simply maintaining its mass. However, even when you were an infant, during which your body was engaged in its most rapid growth period, your need for building material was less than that of fuel.

Nutrients as Regulatory Agents

Regulatory nutrients, as the name indicates, help to regulate the normal chemical reactions of the body. These nutrients, though very important, are typically needed in very small amounts.

Now we can understand why macronutrients (carbohydrates, protein, and fat) form the bulk of the food on your plate — they are burned for energy, and to a lesser extent, used as building material. On the other hand, the micronutrients (vitamins, minerals, and phytonutrients) are needed in very small amounts because they are typically used for their regulatory functions, and therefore are not "used up" as fast.

Filling Up on Fuel

Though the body can burn all three macronutrients for energy, carbohydrates are the primary fuel. Fats are an important secondary fuel, and under certain conditions can have center stage. Either way, carbohydrates and fats are the dynamic duo for providing the body with the bulk of our daily calories.

In other words, the bulk of your calories on any given day will likely come from carbohydrates and/or fat. What about protein? As mentioned in chapter 1, the burning of protein for energy is kept to a minimum, because doing so creates toxicity, leading to serious long-term consequences. This should be taken into consideration by those who want to lose weight by going on a very high protein diet. This issue will be explored more deeply later in the book.

Toxins and Medicine

Now that we understand the three fundamental ways that the body uses nutrients, we can also understand toxins and medicine. Nutrients *maintain* our health. Toxins *disrupt* our health. Medicine helps to *restore* health. For example, pumpkin seeds have chemical agents that help get rid of worms.

Granted, there are instances when the line between nutrient and medicine may be blurred. However, to use medicinal products wisely, we should be mindful of this distinction, because the same substance that can serve as medicine can also poison the body, if used improperly, by taking it in excessive amounts, or for too long a period of time.

In addition, substances that clearly act as nutrients in normal concentrations found in whole foods can have toxic or medicinal effects when used in larger concentrations. For example, the mineral zinc serves a number of normal regulatory functions, but it can quickly become toxic if taken in concentrations beyond what we encounter in whole foods. The vitamin C in whole foods also has many important regulatory functions. Beyond that, some healthcare practitioners use very large doses of vitamin C, sometimes intravenously, to help overcome serious pathologies.

When we understand the distinction between the purely nutritive function of food and its possible medicinal functions, we are less likely to misuse foods and supplements. We understand that any medicine should be used conservatively, so as to avoid toxic side effects.

Individuals who unbalance themselves with food or supplements are typically trying to drug themselves, whether they are doing it for recreational (mood altering) purposes or purely medicinal purposes. Such disruption is more likely when using extracted chemicals (such as vitamins and minerals), compared to whole foods, because the isolated nutrients have been removed from their natural matrix, and concentrated to levels the body normally does not encounter in whole foods.

Even if the toxic effect of a given substance is negligible, imbalances are likely to occur, if we place too much emphasis on selecting food for its medicinal value, because we are more likely to deprive ourselves of nutrients that we would normally receive when we eat to simply nourish the body.

In other words, for optimum health, the rule of thumb is to select foods based on their nutritive virtues. The more precisely we fulfill the body's nutritional needs, the less we have to be concerned about using medicine, natural or otherwise. The simplest and most effective way to fulfill your body's nutritional needs is to base your diet on a variety of fresh whole foods.

A Closer Look at Regulation

Regulation is all about metabolism — a word that is misunderstood as often as it is used. Metabolism simply refers to the sum of all chemical reactions in the body. Though metabolism is vast and complex, there is an underlying simplicity. Our metabolism either has to do with breaking down or building up molecules. Examples include the burning of carbohydrates for energy, and the assemblage of proteins to build and maintain the body.

All of this breaking down and building up of molecules must be carefully regulated. Micronutrients (vitamins, minerals, and phytonutrients) are the champs of regulation. However, this should not be interpreted to mean that macronutrients (carbohydrates, fats, and proteins) have no regulatory functions. They do indeed, but their most obvious functions are that of fuel and building material.

Among the many regulatory roles, three that are particularly significant are those of antioxidants, enzymes and hormones.

- **Antioxidants** are chemicals that neutralize free radicals in the body. Free radical damage is a major cause of aging and degeneration. Free radical damage has been associated with such conditions as arthritis, hair loss, cardiovascular disease, cancer, and wrinkling of skin.[51] Some vitamins and minerals and many phytonutrients have antioxidant activity. Fruits and vegetables are the best sources of antioxidants.
- **Enzymes** are proteins that speed up the chemical reactions of the body. All living organisms make their own enzymes. Regarding diet, most authors acknowledge that some of the enzymes found in foods are valuable in various ways. However, food enzymes are quickly destroyed when heated beyond physiological temperatures (above 115 degrees Fahrenheit), which means that in order to benefit from food-derived enzymes, foods must be consumed raw.
- **Hormones** are chemicals that play important regulatory roles in the body. They often work by regulating enzymes. Though the body manufactures all of its own hormones, some plants have chemicals that have direct hormone-like effects. Also, the types of foods we eat can have a profound effect on hormone production in the body.

What about Water?

We generally do not think of water as a nutrient because it is not burned for energy or used as building material. Nor can it be said to have regulatory functions, as do enzymes, hormones, and antioxidants. However, the countless chemical reactions that make up our metabolism must occur within a watery environment. For this reason, water is indispensable to life and is, in fact, the single most abundant chemical in the body. Therefore, the study of nutrition should include a thoughtful look at our water consumption.

Unless you have a well and a great filtering system, tap water is not ideal, since it is probably chlorinated, fluoridated, and contains industrial pollutants. Regarding diet, the higher our consumption of concentrated foods, or foods that have a relatively high toxic residue, the more water we should drink. In fact, eating foods with a high toxic load makes us thirty because the body is trying to dilute the poisons. This is why salty foods make us thirsty. Of course, the sodium in the salt is an essential nutrient, but it quickly becomes toxic (and therefore triggers thirst) when consumed in amounts higher than what we find in whole foods.

Likewise, we need to drink less water if the diet includes an abundance of high-water-content foods that also have low toxic residue. For example, if your diet consists mostly of cooked grains, beans, and meat, you should drink a substantial amount of water. However, the need to drink water is greatly reduced if your diet consists mostly or entirely of fresh and raw fruits and vegetables. In fact, the water content of most juicy fruit exceeds that of the human body, and therefore has a naturally cleansing and "flushing" effect. Furthermore, such water has been cleansed by the root system of the plant, which is the best filtering system known to us.

It is best to drink more water in the earlier part of the day. This is when the body is most actively involved in cleansing and elimination. In fact, drinking some water upon rising is a good idea because it hydrates the body and gently stimulates the internal organs. However, during a meal, water should be minimized, because it dilutes the digestive juices, and tempts us to eat faster and chew less, leading to indigestion. Therefore, drink water up to about 30 minutes before a meal, and then wait at least one hour after a meal.

Chapter 3
The Nutrients

This chapter has quite a bit of technical information — some of which is not absolutely essential if your bottom line is to just discover your ideal diet. You can certainly learn to eat healthfully without learning the details regarding how the body uses protein, carbohydrates, fats, etc. — just like you can drive your car without knowing how it works. However, the more you know about your car's innards, the better you are at maintaining it, and making adjustments to improve performance and extending its life — without having to be so dependent on a mechanic.

With regard to our nutritional requirements, protein is the nutrient that has typically gotten most of the attention (and virtually all the respect) since the early 20th century. In comparison, the other two macronutrients (carbohydrates and fats) have been treated as second-class citizens.

In fact, as described in chapter 9, advocates of some diets often vilify carbohydrates or fats. They sometimes resort to carbohydrate-bashing, or fat-bashing, as a way of promoting their respective ideas. Nonetheless, an important key for effectively navigating through the sea of diets, is a solid understanding of the roles of carbohydrates and fats. Therefore, this chapter gives close attention to carbohydrates and fats. I certainly do not minimize the importance of having adequate protein in the diet, but rather endeavor to place it in proper perspective.

Carbohydrates

Your typical meal will contain all three macronutrients. However, regardless of their relative amounts, your body will tend to burn carbohydrates first, fats secondly, and proteins last.

Not surprisingly, carbohydrates are the main feature in most traditional diets. In recent years, however, there has been a wave of low-carb diets, which challenge the high-carb approach. Consequently, the average health seeker can become confused. Much of that confusion is cleared away by simply understanding the basics about carbohydrates, and how they dance in the body with fat and protein.

The following chart shows the standard classification of nutritionally significant carbohydrates:

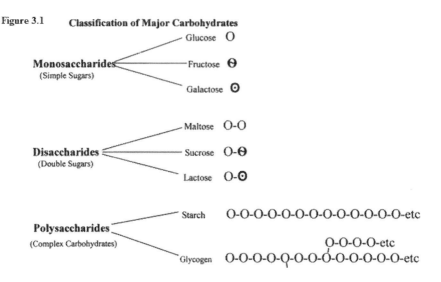

It is not as complicated as it looks. To understand the role of carbohydrates in the body, the three main terms to remember are *sugars, simple sugars,* and *complex carbohydrates* Once you have a clear understanding of these three, the rest is surprisingly easy.

Sugars

The word "sugar" is often used in a way that implies it is just a single substance. That is where the confusion often starts with carbohydrates. The above chart clearly shows that we routinely consume several types of sugars. A sugar is any carbohydrate that easily dissolves in water, and typically tastes sweet.

Sugars come in two varieties: **simple sugars** and **double sugars**. A look at the above chart shows why they have been so named. The chart shows that a simple sugar consists of one relatively small molecule. This is nutritionally significant because the small size allows simple sugars to easily pass from the digestive tract and into the blood without first having to be broken down (digested).

In contrast, a double sugar consists of two simple sugar molecules bonded together. Therefore, double sugars do require digestion through the action of enzymes. Here is a description of the simple and double sugars we tend to consume on a regular basis:

- **Glucose** is our blood sugar. It is abundant in fruits and, to a lesser extent, tender young vegetables.
- **Fructose** is found in many fruits, hence its name.
- **Sucrose** is the sugar you buy in the supermarket in the five-pound bag.
- **Lactose** is found in milk. It is a double sugar, which must be digested. However, many individuals do not have an adequate amount of the enzyme for digesting lactose. The undigested lactose remains in the intestines and is broken down by microbes, resulting in gas. Such individuals are said to be *lactose intolerant*. About 70% of humans have some degree of lactose intolerance, which some dietary authors regard as a sign that milk is not a "natural" food for humans.

Natural and Refined Sugars

Digestion uses up a lot of energy. Therefore, by consuming some nutrients in a "pre-digested" form, such as the simple sugars found in fruits, the body conserves its resources, which can then be used for other purposes, such as powering the immune system and regeneration. This is why athletes often report a dramatic improvement in performance when they start using fruit as a major source of fuel. The fruit does not "give" them more energy, but rather allows the body to *conserve* energy. On the down side, such quick absorption of the sugars can overwhelm the body's ability to process them, leading to blood sugar fluctuations and other issues. A simple way to avoid this problem is to get your sugars in whole foods. The sugars found in fresh fruit come with all of the vitamins, minerals, and other nutrients necessary for the body to process those sugars, as well as fiber to slow down the sugar absorption. In fact, a diet that features three servings of fresh fruit per day has been associated with a decreased risk of diabetes.[1] Because refined sugar is so concentrated, it can have drug-like effects that overpower the self-regulating capacity of the body. Like many drugs, refined sugar is capable of producing true addiction.

Overcoming Sugar Addiction

Total abstinence from refined sugar can be part of the solution. However, we must also provide the body with what it actually needs. Perhaps a lack of minerals or lack of exercise contributes to the addiction.

In the case of sugar addiction, there is an element of grace. For most individuals, there is a simple way to mitigate or even eliminate the addiction to sugary processed foods. Every time you crave something sweet, instead of eating the usual concoctions of refined sugar and fat, just eat some delicious fresh fruit.

Nonetheless, there is disagreement among the various authors regarding how much fruit we can safely consume before the sugars become problematic. We will address this issue in more detail later. For now, a good rule of thumb is that most individuals can enjoy fresh whole fruit, either in moderate amounts or large amounts, depending on the person's physiology and lifestyle. On the other hand, fruit juice, dried fruit, and products containing refined sugar, should be eaten sparingly or avoided entirely.

Fresh fruit does not overpower the senses, as do many processed sweets. If your body can benefit from a moderate amount of fruit, you will desire a moderate amount. If you can benefit from an abundance of fruit, you will desire an abundance of it. Yes, it usually is that simple. Just eat all the fruit you want — and pay attention to your instinctual stop signal.

As a point of caution, however, if you have a history of blood sugar issues and sugar addictions, you may want to favor the lower glycemic fruits, such as strawberries, blueberries, and cherries, because they send sugar into the blood relatively slowly. Also, seek out high quality, organic, and tree/vine ripened fruit. Eat it slowly with no blending or mixing. This way, your brain has the best possible chance of giving you a good clear stop-signal when your body has had enough.

Complex Carbohydrates

A complex carbohydrate consists of many simple sugars strung together, like beads on a string. The nutritionally significant complex carbohydrates are starch and glycogen.

- **Starch** is the most common example of a complex carbohydrate. A starch molecule consists of many glucose molecules strung together, as shown in figure 3.1. Rich sources of starch include grains, legumes, potatoes, and winter squash. Moderately starchy vegetables include kale, broccoli, and cauliflower. Other green leafy vegetables, such as lettuce, spinach, and collards have smaller amounts. When we digest starch, we break down each starch molecule — like separating the individual pearls in a necklace. The glucose released from the starch is burned for energy by our cells. Any surplus is stored as glycogen.

- **Glycogen** is the storage-form of glucose. However, the body can store only a limited amount, because doing so requires a lot of water. This fact allows us to understand why low-carb diets trigger rapid weight loss in the first few days. When we severely restrict the consumption of carbohydrates, the body quickly uses up its glycogen reserves and therefore loses the 2-6 pounds of water associated with the glycogen.

Fabulous Fiber

Fiber is an indigestible complex carbohydrate. Virtually all plants contain fiber. Here are the major health benefits of plant fiber:

- The fiber that coats grains, such as wheat, is called *bran*. Since it has a course texture, it can vigorously "scrub" the walls of the intestines. However, for that same reason, too much can be irritating, and large amounts can actually cause intestinal bleeding in some sensitive individuals.
- The soft fiber in fruit is called *pectin*. It is a form of *soluble fiber*, meaning that it can absorb water and bulk up and quickly move things out of the intestines, which is essential for maintaining a clean and healthy digestive system. Since it is soft, it can be consumed in large amounts without being irritating.
- In addition to physically sweeping the intestines clean, fiber acts like a sponge that absorbs toxins, so they cannot pass into the blood.
- Soluble fiber binds to excess cholesterol in the gut so it does not get absorbed into the blood. Increase in dietary fiber has been shown to lower cholesterol levels.
- Soluble fiber is a source of food for beneficial bacteria in the intestines.
- Fiber slows down the rate at which glucose and other sugars enter the blood, which helps to stabilize blood sugar.

- Fiber promotes weight loss. The added bulk provides a feeling of fullness that prevents overeating high-calorie foods. However, someone who starts eating more fruits and vegetables to lose weight might notice an initial "weight gain" due to the extra fiber and water moving though the intestines. Consequently, they might become discouraged, unless they understand what is actually happening.

Fats and Oils

"Lipids" is the term used by chemists to designate all substances we commonly recognize as solid fats and liquid oils. However, the word "fats" rolls off the tongue so easily that most authors frequently use it in a casual sort of way, which includes both solid fats and liquid oils.

Because of their complexity, the solid fats and liquid oils we consume can be a major source of dietary confusion. The information that follows is probably the most technical part of this book. However, if you are willing to plow through the next several pages, your reward will be the ability to finally understand the role of fats and oils in the diet, as well as giving you the ability to effectively apply the information in making your food choices. If you wish to bypass most of the technical information, you may skip to the end of the fat section, which provides a point-by-point guide to eating fats healthfully.

The Function of Fats

- Our body cells burn fats for energy. Body fat is how we store energy for future use, because it packs twice the calories as the equivalent amount of carbohydrates or protein. In other words, fat allows us to store more fuel in less space.
- The same fat that serves as stored fuel also serves as padding and thermal insulation for the delicate organs.
- Fats are used to manufacture some hormones, such as testosterone and estrogen.
- A certain amount of fat in the diet is needed to allow for proper absorption of some vitamins, minerals, and phytonutrients.
- Some fats are especially important for maintaining a healthy nervous system. The brain is very fatty!

The Problems with Fats

Most of the public attention about fats centers around three topics:
- Cholesterol and triglycerides in the blood.
- Saturated and unsaturated fats in the diet.
- Omega-3 and omega-6 oils in the diet.

Perhaps you have already encountered these terms. Perhaps you are confused by them. If so, you need not be embarrassed. Confusion about fats is quite common, even among health professionals. We can bring some clarity and cohesion to this otherwise slippery subject by first looking at the various types of fats found in the body. The diagram below is the officially recognized classification system, showing how the various types of fats are related to each other.

Figure 3.2 Classsification of Lipids

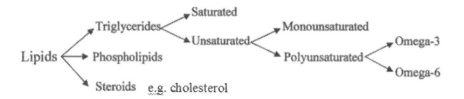

Cholesterol and Triglycerides

Looking at the above chart, the three main types of lipids are triglycerides, steroids, and phospholipids. Of the three, phospholipids are the ones that most people do not know about, because they are the least problematical of the three. However, they are very important, because one of their functions is to prevent other fats from clogging up the body.

The main issue with fats is that they tend to repel water. In that regard, phospholipids are like the diplomats of the biochemical world, allowing other fats to mix with the watery environment of the body. They, literally, work like soap, allowing other fat molecules, such as cholesterol and triglycerides, to mingle with water molecules.

Cholesterol is the most common example of a group of fats called steroids. Since cholesterol is solid and highly insoluble in water, it can easily clump up and clog our tissues. Nonetheless, the liver makes quite a bit of it because it carries out a number of important functions, such as serving as raw material for the manufacture of some hormones, as well as vitamin D. To safely transport cholesterol, it is combined with phospholipids, but that is not enough. Cholesterol is also combined with protein. These complexes exist in two major forms: low density lipoproteins (LDL) and high-density lipoproteins (HDL). When you have your cholesterol levels checked through a blood test, the report you get back makes a distinction between HDL and LDL.

LDL is simplistically but erroneously called "bad cholesterol" and HDL is called "good cholesterol," because LDL is more likely to accumulate in the walls of arteries, while HDL is more likely to stay suspended in the body fluids. However, both have important roles to play in the body, they simply must be kept at their proper levels.

Triglycerides form the bulk of the animal fats and vegetable oils we eat. As with cholesterol, we should have a certain amount of triglycerides in the blood, not too much and not too little. Measuring the level of blood triglycerides is important for assessing cardiovascular health. To understand the importance of triglycerides and the health problems that can arise from having too little or too much, let us first consider the two major types: saturated and unsaturated.

Saturated and Unsaturated Fats

Triglycerides are composed mostly of smaller molecules called fatty acids. "Saturated" and "unsaturated" simply refer to two types of fatty acids. Looking at the two pictures below, we can easily see the difference between saturated and unsaturated fatty acids:

The saturated fatty acid is completely filled or "saturated" with hydrogen atoms (H). This feature makes the molecule straight, allowing neighboring triglyceride molecules to stack up with each other. Therefore, they can easily stick together, like Velcro, to form a solid fat. In contrast, the unsaturated fatty acid has "bare spots" where hydrogen is missing. This feature causes the molecule to be kinked, which makes it more difficult to stick to surrounding molecules — like wrinkled Velcro. The lack of cohesion results in the formation of a liquid oil, rather than a solid fat.

Figure 3.3: Saturated Fatty Acid

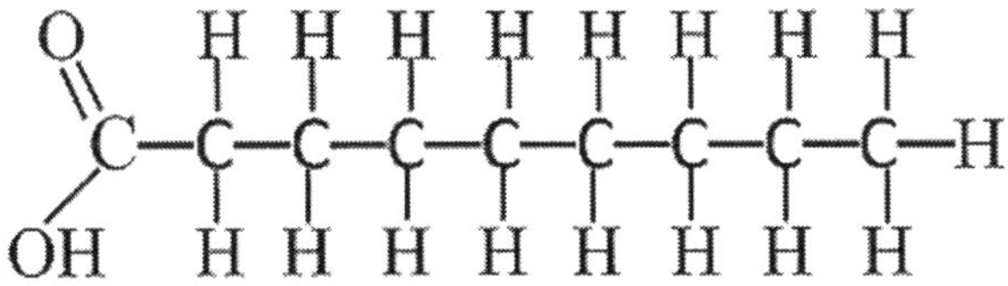

Figure 3.4 Mono-unsaturated Fatty Acid

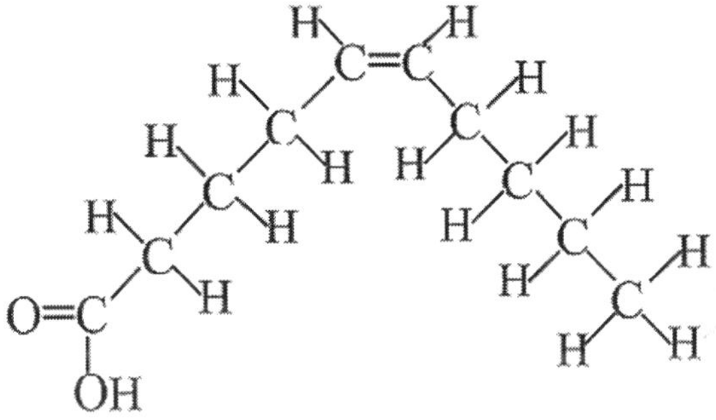

In addition, the specific unsaturated fatty acid shown above may be said to be *monounsaturated*, which means it has only one bare spot. Consequently, it is only moderately kinked. Therefore, though the molecules are not straight enough to form solid fats, the liquid oils they produce tend to be rather thick and easily turn solid if cooled down a bit below room temperature. For example, olive oil consists mostly of monounsaturated fats, and is about 14% saturated. This is why it is very thick at room temperature and turns solid when refrigerated.

In contrast, *polyunsaturated* fatty acids have multiple bare spots along the chain, resulting in a very kinked structure. Like badly wrinkled Velcro, these chains do not stick together well at all, and therefore produce relatively thin oils that remain liquid even when placed in a very cold refrigerator.

The great fluidity of polyunsaturated oils makes them easier to handle by the body because they are more easily transported through the body's watery environment. This same feature also makes them extremely important for a number of vital body functions, especially that of the brain and immune system. These functions may be best understood by considering two types of polyunsaturated oils that are of special importance to us: omega-3 and omega-6.

Omega-3 and Omega-6 Oils

Omega-3 and omega-6 are two types of polyunsaturated oils that must be kept in the right proportion for the body to remain healthy. A vast variety of moderate to very serious health issues stem from inadequate amounts or improper ratios of these two oils. Until recently, imbalances of these two oils had received little attention. However, their impact is no less important than that of cholesterol and saturated fats. In fact, the cardiovascular issues that were once totally blamed on saturated fats and cholesterol now appear to also be affected by an imbalance of omega-3 and omega-6.

Omega-3 fats are found in nuts, seeds, and animal products, especially fish and eggs. Omega-6 oils are found in peanut oil, soybean oil, corn oil, safflower oil, nuts, and seeds. Many animal products, such as beef, pork, dairy, and some fish are also high in omega-6. Most individuals eating the usual civilized diet have inadequate levels of omega-3 oils and too much omega-6, which contributes to pain, inflammation, depression, cardiovascular problems, and other forms of degeneration.

Omega-3 oils from plant foods are used to make two other critically important omega-3 oils: EPA (eicosapentanoic acid) and DHA (docosahexanoic acid). One serious consequence of having too much omega-6 is that the body has a hard time converting dietary omega-3 oils into EPA and DHA.

Furthermore, even when the ratio of dietary omega-3 and omega-6 in the diet is proper, some individuals may still have a hard time making adequate amounts of EPA and DHA, and therefore depend on food sources, such as eggs and fish. This could be one reason some individuals seem to require animal products, while others seem to thrive for many years on a vegan or near vegan diet, without supplementation with EPA and DHA.

DHA is particularly important for brain function. About 30% of the fat in the brain is DHA. Perhaps this is why fish has traditionally been known as "brain food." Lack of DHA has been linked to depression, aggression, reduced intelligence, sleep problems, alcoholism, and bipolar disorder.

The Four Major Dietary Issues with Fats

Volumes have been written about the potential problems with ingested fats. However, from a practical standpoint, we can point to four major issues:

- **Too Much Cholesterol and Saturated Fat.** Cholesterol and saturated fats are solid at body temperature. (The exceptions are the short-chained saturated fats, such as butter, palm oil, and coconut oil, which are solid at room temperature, but melt at body temperature). Because saturated fats are usually solid at body temperature, they tend to stiffen cells' membranes, which can interfere with the cells' ability to communicate with their environment. This is especially detrimental for the brain and immune system. In addition, high levels of saturated fats and cholesterol have been linked to insulin resistance.[2,3] What about cardiovascular health? Yes, high levels of cholesterol and saturated fats seem to be risk factors. Also, recent evidence does show that saturated fats tend to make arteries less elastic.[4] However, the connection between saturated fats, cholesterol, and cardiovascular disease is not as simplistic as once believed.[5,6] Unfortunately, the subtleties of this issue require a detailed explanation that would make this section even more technical than it already is. For the reader who is interested, Appendix D offers a more detailed explanation of this issue. The bottom line is this: lowering cholesterol and saturated fat (and doing nothing else) is not likely to decrease your risk of cardiovascular disease.[7,8]

- **Too Much Omega-6 Oils.** Excessive amount of these oils results in greater likelihood of pain, inflammation, and various degenerative diseases. To complicate matters, the excess of omega-6 is often accompanied by a lack of omega-3.
- **Partially Hydrogenated Oils and Trans-fats.** Liquid vegetable oils are artificially solidified by introducing hydrogen into unsaturated oils. This is how margarine and shortening are made. The problem with artificially solidified fats is that our cells do not utilize them as well as the original oil, resulting in a wide variety of problems. In addition, the altered fatty acids are not completely hydrogenated, but rather *partially* hydrogenated, which means that part of the molecule is left unsaturated. Such altered molecules are called trans-fats. They have been linked to high cholesterol, cardiovascular disease, diabetes, cancer, ADD (attention deficit disorder), and ADHD (attention deficit and hyperactivity disorder). Some trans-fats occur naturally, but will increase when the foods are exposed to heat and light. However, the highest levels, by far, are found in partially hydrogenated vegetable oils. For example, the level of trans-fats in margarine is about 100 times higher than that of eggs. The reduction of trans-fats in the diet has been shown to help with ADD, ADHD, MS, and Parkinson's disease.[9]

- **Oxidized Oils.** This issue gets the least attention compared to the other three, but it is ultimately of equal importance to our health. Fats can oxidize (become rancid) when exposed to air, heat or light. When they do so, they become toxic. For example, one of the major issues with dietary cholesterol has to do with the fact that some of it has been oxidized through cooking and processing. The oxidized cholesterol can irritate the inner lining of arteries, which, in turn, can lead to plaque formation.[10] However, oxidized fat *of any kind* can do this! In fact, overall, polyunsaturated oils might be even more problematical in this regard, because they are much more vulnerable to oxidation than saturated fats and cholesterol. *The more unsaturated the oil, the more sensitive it is to oxidation.* For the same reason, omega-3 oils are more vulnerable than omega-6. Likewise, of all the omego-3 oils, EPA and DHA (especially the latter) are the most sensitive to oxidation — simply because they are the most unsaturated. The fishy smell of fish is due to oxidized omega-3 oils (mostly DHA) — which are quite toxic. In contrast, live or freshly caught fish do not have that odor. Furthermore, when these oils are extracted from whole foods, they are separated from their protective antioxidant matrix, subjected to heat and light, and sit for a long time in a warehouse or brightly lit store. Therefore, some oxidation is likely to occur.

Guidelines for Eating Fats

- Favor whole-food fats instead of extracted oils.
- If you buy extracted oils, use them sparingly and make sure they are fresh. Buy them in small amounts so you use them up in a timely manner. Keep them refrigerated.
- To minimize the long-term detrimental effects of oxidization, favor raw fats. Cook the fatty foods when you need to; eat them raw when you can.
- If you cook or bake with oil, favor the heavier oils, such as coconut oil, palm oil, and olive oil — in moderation! Coconut and palm oil are saturated, and olive oil is mostly monounsaturated. Therefore, these oils are less reactive under heat, compared to those oils that are rich in polyunsaturates.

- Be moderate with dietary saturated fats and cholesterol.
- Eliminate partially hydrogenated vegetable oils (trans-fats). Read the label.
- Balance the omega-6 and omega-3 oils. The ideal ratio is about 2:1 in favor of omega-6 (or 1:1 depending on who you ask). The typical diet that is high in grains, vegetables oils, and grain-fed meat might be around 20:1 or 30:1 in favor of omega-6! A healthier ratio is provided by a diet rich in fruits and vegetables, while featuring the appropriate amount of other foods, such as fish, grass-fed meats, nuts, and seeds.

Protein

The dry weight of the body is mostly protein. When this was first discovered in the early 20th century, the scientists and health care practitioners of the day jumped to an erroneous conclusion — they assumed protein should be the dominant feature of the diet. That conclusion quickly found its way to the general public, where it eventually became so deeply entrenched that it persists to the present day, even though subsequent research has clearly shown otherwise.

To understand why we do not need large quantities of protein, let us consider what happens to it after we eat it. Protein is first digested into smaller molecules called amino acids. Then, our body cells reassemble the amino acids into our own proteins, such as those that make up muscles, bones, tendons, ligaments, hair, nails, blood vessels, and vital organs.

In other words, the body uses protein primarily as building material. Furthermore, the body does not simply discard worn out proteins, but rather "recycles" them — their constituent amino acids are salvaged and used again. Therefore, the amount of protein that is lost, and must be replaced through food, is actually quite small.

Protein Requirements

The official requirements for dietary protein are about 56 grams for the average adult males and 44 for females. This generally translates into 10-15% of daily calories coming from protein. Since the actual dietary requirements are low, the main emphasis should not be on quantity but quality. A so-called high-quality protein is one having all essential amino acids in the proper proportion to suit our needs. In general, protein from animal foods is considered high quality because its amino acid profile closely resembles that of our own proteins. In contrast, a given plant protein may be deficient in one or more essential amino acids. To get all essential amino acids from plants, variety is the key.

Protein Toxicity

Though the various diets described in chapter 9 often disagree as to whether carbohydrates or fats should provide the bulk of calories, virtually all of them agree that protein should not be the primary source. High protein diets have been linked to osteoporosis, hip fractures, cancer, Alzheimer's disease, cardiovascular disease, kidney damage, and accelerated aging of the body. The reason? Surplus protein is toxic. The amino acids that are not used as building material or to make other substances are burned for energy, resulting in the production of ammonia, which is so extremely toxic that the liver converts it into urea (and perhaps uric acid). Therefore, we should get ample dietary protein to allow for growth and maintenance, but not so much as to force the body to burn the excess. Protein toxicity is described in more detail in chapter 5.

Vitamins, Minerals and Phytonutrients

We can best understand these nutrients by first remembering that they are collectively called *micronutrients*, which calls attention to the fact that we need them in minuscule amounts. In contrast, carbohydrates, fats and protein are called *macronutrient*s, because we need them in larger amounts.

We need larger amounts of macronutrients because we burn them for energy or use them as building material, while having less obvious roles in regulation. On the other hand, vitamins, minerals, and phytonutrients have no obvious roles as fuel or building material, but rather are *all* about regulation. For example, vitamins and minerals are important for activating enzymes, while many phytonutrients serve as antioxidants.

Until the early 20th century, micronutrients received very little attention. They are easy to overlook because, for most of recorded history, serious deficiencies were not that common. Since our ancestors ate mostly fresh whole foods, dangerously low levels of vitamins, minerals, and phytonutrients were unlikely. Humans were more likely to die from starvation (lack calories) before they fell from micronutrient deficiencies. All that changed as more people ate refined or heavily processed foods, which pack on the calories, while seriously reducing the vitamins, minerals, and phytonutrients.

Vitamins
- Vitamin A – retinol
- Vitamin B1 – thiamine
- Vitamin B2 – riboflavin
- Vitamin B3 – niacin
- Vitamin B5 – pantothenic acid
- Vitamin B6 – pyridoxine
- Vitamin B12 – cobolamin (methylcobolamin or cyanocobolamin)
- Folate
- Vitamin C – ascorbic acid
- Vitamin D – calciferol
- Vitamin E – tocopherol

B vitamins and vitamin C are water-soluble. They are measured in milligrams. Vitamins A, D, E and K are fat-soluble. They are measured in international units (IU).

B Vitamins

B vitamins are of special interest because their deficiency is what alerted scientists to the existence of vitamins, in general. In the latter 19th century, polished rice was introduced into the Asian diet. Polished rice has no bran, which makes it more appealing and easier to cook. However, this practice was followed by a dramatic rise in the death rate from a disease called beriberi, which eventually was found to be caused by severe B vitamin deficiency.

B vitamins were eventually found to be important for the nervous system, skin, hair, eyes, and digestive system. Symptoms of deficiency include fatigue, depression, constipation, and gray hair. B vitamins are found in whole grains, fruits, and vegetables. Vitamin B_{12} is the only B vitamin that is not readily available in plant foods, but is produced by soil and intestinal bacteria. The largest concentrations of B_{12} are found in animal products, but modest amounts are also found in mushrooms and sea vegetation.

The role of intestinal bacteria in providing B_{12} has not been well established, however, animal studies suggest these bacteria may be an important source. For example, researchers were not able to induce B_{12} deficiencies in other primates by dietary restriction of B_{12}. Instead, researchers were able to induce B_{12} deficiencies by giving animals antibiotics![11]

Vitamin C

Vitamin C is another vitamin with an interesting history. The first clue to its importance was the death of thousands of sailors, centuries ago, from a disease called scurvy, in which the individual experiences extreme bone fragility and massive bleeding. Eventually, a British doctor discovered that giving sailors oranges, lemons or limes prevented scurvy — that is why British sailors were later called "Limeys." However, it was not until the 1930s that scurvy was discovered to be actually caused by a serious deficiency of vitamin C. This vitamin is essential for the production of collagen, the main protein that holds together the many tissues of the body — including bones and blood vessels. No wonder sailors were dying from uncontrolled bleeding and crumbling bones!

How Much Vitamin C Do We Really Need?

In addition to human studies, a look at the rest of the animal kingdom suggests a much higher need for this vitamin than the 75-90 milligrams given by government health authorities.[12] Most animals make their own vitamin C. How much do they make? They produce at least ten times the official RDI.[13]

Humans are among the few animals that must get vitamin C from food. Monkeys and apes in the wild that get vitamin C entirely from food, do so in amounts that are 10-20 times the RDI for humans.[11] For example, gorillas get 5,000-10,000 milligrams of vitamin C per day!

Like other animals in the wild, gorillas do not suffer from obesity, cardiovascular disease, or blood sugar issues. However gorillas in captivity have been known to develop these conditions, as well as die prematurely for no apparent reason. Was it a lack of vitamin C? Studies on gorillas in captivity showed an improvement in health when given the levels of vitamin C they would normally receive in the wild.

Human studies have shown a link between low levels of vitamin C and a number of health issues, such as high cholesterol, cardiovascular disease, bleeding gums, bruising, strokes, excess fat storage, asthma, greater susceptibility to respiratory infections, such as the flu, low energy, fatigue, rapid aging of tissues, and cancer.

> How much vitamin C should we really get for optimum health? Difficult to say. However, It is reasonable to suggest that optimal levels are similar to those observed in wild animals. These so-called "mega-doses" have been shown to protect against some of above-mentioned pathological conditions.

Minerals

While vitamins can be broken down through cooking, minerals are not, because they are elements pulled out of the earth. However, that means the depletion of minerals from soil will leave the plant mineral deficient as well. This is one of the concerns about modern farming, which progressively strips minerals from soil.

The major minerals in the body include:
- **Calcium:** Dairy, dark leafy greens, figs, oranges, sesame seeds, and fish.
- **Magnesium:** Vegetables, fruits, seeds, and nuts.
- **Sodium:** Seafood, meat, poultry, beets, carrots, celery, tomatoes, Swiss chard.
- **Potassium:** Virtually all fruits and vegetables.

Trace minerals consist of about 65 minerals, such as chromium, zinc, iron, and selenium. They are needed in much lesser amounts, but are equally important.

Like vitamins, minerals are needed to activate enzymes. They are also important for establishing the proper acid/alkaline balance (pH) of the body. Some minerals, such as sulfur, phosphorous, iodine, and chlorine, tend to acidify the body. Other minerals, such as calcium, sodium, potassium, and magnesium, tend to alkalize the body. For optimum health, it is recommended that we eat a diet consisting of about 80% alkalizing foods and 20% acid-forming foods. Most fruits and vegetables tend to be alkalizing, while animal products, grains, nuts, and seeds tend to be acidifying.

Phytonutrients

The term phytonutrients includes a broad category of plant-derived nutrients having many regulatory functions, such as serving as antioxidants. Fruits and vegetables having high phytonutrient content are typically colorful: red, orange, yellow, purple, and deep green. There are many thousands of phytonutrients. A tomato has about 10,000. Two of the best-known categories of phytonutrients are **flavonoids** and **carotenoids**.

Carotenoids include beta-carotene, which the body converts into vitamin A. Flavonoids are closely associated with vitamin C. They are found in all the same foods that provide vitamin C. The combination of vitamin C and flavonoids is important for reducing inflammation, fighting infections, and building collagen. Some flavonoids seem to have a beneficial effect on brain chemistry, promoting positive mental and emotional states.

Phytonutrients, like most of the vitamins, are damaged when heated to cooking temperatures. Since it is virtually impossible to get all of them in supplement form, individuals who eat predominantly cooked food are likely to be deficient in phytonutrients. This might also account for some of the reported benefits of a totally or mostly raw diet.

Chapter 4
The Food Groups

Any whole food has a variety of nutrients. However, for our needs, a given food may be a rich source of some nutrients, while being deficient in others. Therefore, variety is important if we want to get all the nutrients we need.

Grains

Grains form the basis of diets in most parts of the world. Grains include wheat, barley, rye, corn, rice, oats, and millet. The tough outer covering of the grain is made of a coarse fiber called bran, which is also rich in vitamins and minerals. For example, rice bran is used as a source of B vitamins.

The inside of the grain is rich in starch. Most grains also have a significant amount of protein. The major protein found in grains is called gluten. White bread and pasta are made of wheat that has been refined, which means that the bran (and most of the vitamins and minerals) has been removed.

Though whole grains are usually inexpensive, convenient, and provide a goodly amount of calories, protein, and micronutrients, they have some features that necessitate a degree of moderation, or even elimination for some individuals. Here are the main points to consider:

- Grains have protease inhibitors, which can inhibit protein digestion.
- They contain phytate, which, in high levels, has been said to inhibit the absorption of some minerals (zinc, iron, calcium, magnesium) by the body. However, this has been questioned.
- They are high in calories, mostly in the form of starch, which effectively increases with cooking, because it becomes more bioavailable.
- Since the caloric content is high, a diet that provides the bulk of calories from grains can lead to deficiencies in vitamins, minerals, and phytonutrients. This becomes even more problematical if the grains are refined — which is often the case. This is why the sudden introduction

of refined rice and wheat in Asia in the nineteenth century was followed with a sharp increase in a potentially fatal disease called beriberi.
- Since cooked grains tend to be bland, flavor enhancers and fats are generally added, which can promote overconsumption.
- Wheat, rye, and barley have high levels of gluten, which can trigger allergic reactions in some individuals. In general, non-hybridized grains are easier to digest and are less allergenic than heavily hybridized grains. If the gluten sensitivity is severe enough, it is diagnosed as celiac disease.

Tips for Healthy Grain Eating

- Favor whole grain products, preferably organically grown.
- Eat grains in the amounts appropriate to your body's ability to utilize them.
- Even if you handle grains well, don't just fill up on them. Leave room for vegetables.
- In addition to the usual grains, like wheat, corn, and rice, include the lesser known but nutritionally more balanced (and less allergenic) grains, such as millet, amaranth, and quinoa. Also, buckwheat is an excellent grain substitute.
- Avoid genetically modified (GMO) grains, which, like other genetically modified foods, may not be as benign as the public has been led to believe. There is still much controversy about this, but that is reason enough to be very cautious and simply avoid them until they have been proven safe, especially when we consider that corn and wheat are widely used.[1,2] Currently most commercially grown wheat and corn in the United States is GMO. Labeling of GMO products is not required, therefore, the way to avoid GMO grains is to buy organic or naturally grown food.
- Look for bread made with sourdough instead of just yeast. In addition to having some yeast, sourdough has bacteria — the same sort of beneficial bacteria that populate our intestines. These bacteria reduce the levels of irritants and antinutrients in grains, as well as producing a number of beneficial byproducts, including B vitamins, amino acids, and lactic acid. The latter discourages the growth of harmful organisms in the digestive tract. When you buy sourdough bread, read the label and make sure that one of the ingredients is *sourdough starter*. Some commercial forms are called "sourdough bread" but are actually yeast bread with other chemicals thrown in to make it taste like sourdough.

Legumes

Legumes include beans, peas, lentils, and peanuts. Since legumes are seeds, they are rich in protein and carbohydrates. Legumes are reputed to have a number of health-giving benefits. The gas associated with legumes is attributed to difficulty in digesting the carbohydrate component. Soaking and sprouting, as done in some traditional diets, reduces the gas, as does cooking. For those who can digest legumes well, these foods are an excellent source of plant-based protein, as well as soluble fiber, minerals, and phytonutrients. However, there are two common legumes that should be closely examined before they are liberally included in the diet: peanuts and soybeans.

Peanuts

Like other legumes, peanuts are high in protein. They are also very high in fat (peanut oil). One of the issues with peanuts is their tendency to trigger allergic reactions. The other issue is the presence of carcinogenic substances, called aflatoxins that accumulate on the surface, mostly due to prolonged storage inside the shell. In light of these two issues, I would advise the health seeker to eat peanuts in moderation or avoid them altogether.

Soybeans

Soy has the highest protein content of any legume. Because it is cheap and versatile, it is widely used. However, there is much controversy about soy in the nutrition world. Here are the main points to consider: The most beneficial forms of soy are the traditional fermented products, such as miso, shoyu (soy sauce), tempeh, and natto. Much of the reliable evidence that links soy to reduction in cancer and heart disease came from Japan, where soy has been traditionally consumed in the form of fermented soy products.

Fermentation makes soy more digestible. For example, fermentation, along with soaking and cooking, reduces the level of the gas-producing carbohydrates. Fermentation reduces the antinutrients (see below) found in soybeans and creates beneficial substances, including vitamins, antioxidants, and enzymes. For example, one of the enzymes found in natto is called nattokinase, which has been found to break down blood clots, thin the blood, and lower blood pressure.

Soybeans that have not been soaked, well cooked, sprouted or fermented contain several substances that are the focal point of controversy, such as allergens, phytate, protease inhibitors, and estrogen like-substances.

Tofu and Other Soy Products

Tofu is an extract of protein found in soybeans. Traditional tofu was often fermented, while most commercial tofu is not. On the positive side, tofu is inexpensive, and eliminates the indigestible carbohydrate that produces gas. However, we should bear in mind that tofu is not a *whole* food. Digesting tofu is not unlike digesting pasteurized cheese or cooked meat, requiring a large output of enzymes.

Other processed unfermented soy products include soy flour, soy lecithin, and textured vegetable protein (TVP). The latter is high in MSG (monosodium glutamate). Some of the health problems encountered by modern vegetarians and vegans may be attributed to the over-consumption of highly processed soy products. In contrast, vegetarian or near vegetarian societies that show good health and longevity, typically consume an abundance of fresh fruits and vegetables, along with whole grains, legumes, and starchy vegetables.

Furthermore, much of the commercially produced soybeans in the United States are genetically modified and sprayed heavily with pesticides and herbicides. In fact, the genetically modified soybeans have been specifically engineered to tolerate larger doses of a certain herbicide, which means that when you eat those beans, you get the double whammy of genetic modification and higher levels of herbicide residue.

Bottom Line on Soy

If you decide to use soy as food, you may want to favor the traditional fermented soy products, made from organically grown soybeans. Such soy is nutritious and has real health benefits. If tofu is appealing to you, eat it in moderation, favor the traditional fermented kind, and combine it with a liberal amount of vegetables and a good source of trace minerals, such as sea vegetation, as done in traditional Asian diets.

Let soy be a modest part of a larger legume repertoire that includes a wide variety of other whole legumes, such as black beans, black-eyed peas, and lentils. Fresh and tender legumes, such as green beans, sweet peas, snow peas, and fava beans are also excellent, and can be eaten cooked or raw. And stay away from any GMO soy, which means get the organic or naturally grown soy.

Fruits

A fruit is the fleshy covering around a seed. Fruits tend to be rich in simple sugars, vitamins, minerals, and antioxidants. Compared to other food groups, they tend to be lowest in fat and protein.

Fruit Is Clean Food

Of all the food groups, fruit is the easiest to digest, and allows for the most efficient cleanup. Here are the reasons::

- It has the highest water content of the food groups.
- It is high in soluble fiber, which absorbs water and provides bulk that keeps the GI tract well-hydrated and clean.
- The soluble fiber absorbs toxins that would otherwise pass into the blood.
- Soluble fiber is soft and easy on the digestive tract, so it can be consumed in large quantities without irritation of the inner lining of the GI tract.
- Fruit has the least toxic residue of all foods (unless it has been heavily sprayed with herbicides and pesticides).
- Since fruit is typically consumed raw, it avoids the added toxic burden that is produced by cooking.
- Fruit provides most of its carbohydrates, protein, and fat in a predigested form. As part of the ripening process, enzymes in the fruit break down starch into glucose, proteins into amino acids, fats into fatty acids and glycerol. Therefore, fruit requires the least amount of energy for digestion and cleanup, thus allowing the body to conserve energy, which can then be used to promote deeper cleansing and regeneration.
- Fruit is tasty and nutritious enough to be consumed as a mono-meal or snack, which optimizes digestion.

Some Fruits of Interest

- **Apples** Contain malic acid, which stimulates cleansing of the liver, and has been shown to be beneficial for individuals with fibromyalgia.
- **Bananas** are very rich in potassium and contain several factors that calm the emotions and lift depression. Fully ripe bananas contain a chemical that inhibits tumor growth, inhibits viral replication, and enhances the immune system.
- **Blueberries** are high in antioxidants, good for heart, brain, and eyes.
- **Strawberries** are high in antioxidants, and rich in xylitol, which may account for strawberries having a reputation for being good for teeth and gums.
- **Red or purple grapes** are high in antioxidants, especially resveratrol, which has been shown to promote cardiovascular health and activates two so-called "anti-aging" genes

- **Prunes** have the highest antioxidant content of any common fruit or vegetable.
- **Pineapples** contain bromelain, an enzyme that digests protein and has been shown to have anti-inflammatory effects.
- **Papaya** contain papain, a protein-digesting enzyme.
- **Watermelon** promotes cleansing of the intestines, liver, and kidneys. It is rich in lycopene, and is reputed to be beneficial for individuals with psoriasis, arthritis, and kidney stones. It also promotes the production of nitric oxide, which protects the inner lining of the blood vessels and helps to lower blood pressure.
- **Figs** are high in calcium and iron. Very cleansing, especially mucus.
- **Pomegranates** are very rich in antioxidants, and help to lower blood pressure. Has been shown in human and animal studies to <u>reverse</u> arterial plaquing.[3]
- **Kiwi fruit** are very rich in enzymes, vitamin C, and lutein. Also rich in vitamin E, folate, and potassium.

Vegetables

The term "vegetables" typically refers to edible roots, stems, and leaves. Some so-called vegetables, such as cucumbers, are fruits, technically. In the language of botany, fruit is simply the soft covering around the seeds. To a botanist, cucumbers, tomatoes, bell peppers, and okra are fruits, but their nutritional profile resembles that of other vegetables, more so than fruit. Fleshy vegetables, such as potatoes and squash, are rich in starch.

Eat Your Vegetables!

Your mother was right. Here is why:
- Vegetables tend to be rich in minerals, which make them good for alkalizing and cleansing the blood.
- Green leafy vegetables tend to be rich in vitamins and phytonutrients, many of which are powerful antioxidants. They protect against inflammation, aging, and degeneration. Yellow and orange vegetables are rich in beta carotene, which the body converts into vitamin A.
- Vegetables provide their wealth of vitamins, minerals, and phytonutrients, while also being very low in calories. This means it is virtually impossible to over-consume vegetables. You can literally fill your

stomach with veggies, while getting just a few hundred calories. For this reason, vegetables are valuable for individuals who want to be moderate with their caloric intake without becoming deficient in essential nutrients. For the same reason, vegetables are essential for individuals on low carb-diets, who eat a lot of animal products, but want to make sure they get their vitamins, minerals, and phytonutrients, while still keeping their consumption of carbohydrate calories relatively low.

Some Vegetables of Interest
- **Carrots** are rich in beta-carotene, which, among other benefits, promotes eye health. They also contain oils that help to eliminate intestinal parasites. They promote cleansing of the liver.
- **Beets** are rich in iron. They promote cleansing of the liver.
- **Dandelion greens** promote cleansing of the liver.
- **Celery** is an excellent source of minerals. Soothing for the nervous system. Helps to lower blood pressure.
- **Broccoli** has essential oils that have anticancer properties. Rich in vitamin K. Rich in sulfur-containing oils, which help detoxify the liver.
- **Kale** has the highest antioxidant content of any vegetable. It is a good source of calcium and iron. Like other dark green leafy vegetables, it promotes cleansing of the liver and blood. Like broccoli, it is rich in sulfur-containing oils.
- **Spinach,** like other dark green leafy vegetables, promotes cleansing of the liver and blood. It is rich in antioxidants and iron.

Nuts and Seeds

From a nutritional standpoint, the foods we classify as nuts and seeds can generally be eaten raw, though roasting is a common practice. They tend to be high in proteins and fats. Many nuts are excellent sources of trace minerals.

Since nuts and seeds tend to be rich in fats, they are best eaten in moderation. Also, their rough texture can irritate the stomach and intestines if eaten in large amounts. They are most nutritious when eaten raw, soaked, and maybe sprouted.

Some Nuts and Seeds of Interest
- **Walnuts** contain about 60 chemicals that are beneficial for the brain.

- **Flax seeds** are good for the intestines, and are an excellent source of omega-3 fatty acids, fiber, and various other beneficial phytonutrients. They promote intestinal motility, and enhance the growth of beneficial bacteria.
- **Pumpkin seeds** are rich in zinc. They are excellent for the reproductive organs, especially the prostate. They also contain oils that help eliminate intestinal worms.
- **Sesame seeds** are an excellent source of trace minerals. The lignins in sesame seeds have many health benefits, such as protecting against free radical damage of DNA, and other forms of free radical damage. They also help to lower cholesterol and reduce inflammation.
- **Almonds** are relatively low in oils and high in protein (compared to other nuts and seeds). According to some sources, they have anticancer properties.
- **Sunflower seeds** are highly nutritious, easy to sprout, and inexpensive.
- **Brazil nuts** are rich in protein, and very rich in selenium. In fact, they are so high in selenium that more than a few per day for extended period of time can lead to selenium toxicity.

Animal Products

Animal products include all foods derived from the bodies of animals, as well as their eggs, milk, and milk products. The term "flesh foods" refers to any edible part of land animals, birds, or fish. The term "meat" generally refers to the muscles of land animals, which might include poultry, depending on whom you ask. The term, "organ meat" includes liver, kidneys, and pancreas. "Red meat" generally refers to the muscles of hoofed animals, most notably beef.

Animal products are rich in protein and fat. A quarter of a pound (four ounces) of beef, chicken or fish provides about 25 grams of protein. The protein in animal products is considered to be of high quality because it closely resembles our own proteins in terms of amino acid profile. By weight, the fat content is typically less than the protein, but in terms of calories, the fat content can actually be higher, because a given amount of fat has over twice the calories as the same amount of protein. Animal-based foods also contain certain nutrients that tend to be lacking or more difficult to get in plant foods, especially DHA, vitamin B_{12}, vitamin D_3, selenium, and zinc.

Here are the reasons to be moderate with animal-based foods:
- The fat portion includes a substantial amount of saturated fat, cholesterol, and some trans-fats.
- The toxic residue tends to be higher compared to plant-based foods. For example, red meat is associated with iron toxicity, which increases the oxidative stress on the body and has been associated with increased cancer rates and oxidation of cholesterol. In Also, flesh food, especially red meat, is high in uric acid, which, among other things, stimulates the body in a manner similar to caffeine. This might be one reason some individuals feel better "right away" when they resume eating red meat.
- Animal products are also subject to contamination, which largely has to do with the dirty farming practices that usually occur on a mass production scale. Salmonella contamination was found in a high percentage of inspected poultry. The routine use of antibiotics in cattle results in the breeding of virulent strains of E. coli. I am personally acquainted with one former poultry inspector who eventually became a vegan, after seeing how commercial poultry and other meats are produced.

The above facts are no reason to totally exclude animal products, but rather to exercise moderation, and buy organic, as with grains and soy products. The good news is that the specific nutrients provided by animal products are so concentrated that we do not have to consume very large amounts of these foods to get the nutritional benefits.

Fish

Fish is the most easily digestible and nutritionally complete flesh food, especially if it is eaten raw as in sushi. In addition to being a good source of protein, fish are high in omega-3 oils and minerals.

Though fish (wild fish, at least) are not subject to the antibiotics and other chemicals used in growing livestock, fish from polluted waters obviously pose a problem. The major concern with fish is the mercury content. In general, big fish that live a long time, such as tuna, have higher mercury content than small fish that have a shorter life cycle. Below is a guide for minimizing mercury exposure from fish, based on government and academic sources:

- *Lowest mercury content:* Salmon, sardines, sole, freshwater catfish, shrimp
- *Limit to once per week*: Orange roughy, sea bass, *red snapper, *flounder, *fresh water bass, *halibut, *fresh tuna
- *Limit to once per month:* *Swordfish, *shark, tilefish, *king mackerel, *marlin

*These fish were found to occasionally have unsafe levels of mercury. The biggest and oldest fish consistently had the highest levels.

Pork, Beef, Poultry, Eggs

Pork leaves the largest toxic residue of the flesh foods and can harbor a swarm of parasitic infections, most notably trichinosis, as well as possibly harboring large amounts of viruses, which are not necessarily eliminated by normal cooking. Pork is also not easy to digest. By thoroughly cooking it at high temperatures (which is necessary to eliminate the parasites), it becomes even more difficult to digest.

Beef tends to be cleaner than pork, because the traditional food of cows (grass) is cleaner than the food consumed by pigs. Grass-fed beef is available in some supermarkets, as well as some farmers markets. Grass-fed beef is substantially better than grain and soy fed beef. In fact, since the corn and soy that is routinely fed to cows is GMO, I would advise individuals who consume beef on a regular basis to avoid commercially raised beef and find good sources of organic grass-fed beef.

Poultry tends to be more digestible than beef and has less saturated fat. Commercially raised chicken is loaded with toxic residue, such as arsenic (found in chicken feed), but free-range chicken and turkey are readily available in some supermarkets, farmers markets, and health food stores.

Eggs are an excellent source of protein, omega-3 oils and fat-soluble vitamins. However, commercial eggs come from factory-raised chickens, which have been raised under extremely unsanitary conditions, are loaded with antibiotics, and are subject to salmonella. Organic eggs are available in health food stores and some supermarkets. They contain higher levels of important fatty acids, especially DHA. The really good organic eggs will have a rich orange yolk and are generally tastier than commercial eggs.

Milk Products

Milk is a mixture of nutrients designed to support the growing baby. It contains protein (mostly casein), sugar (lactose), and fat. It is also loaded with vitamins and minerals. It is especially rich in calcium. The protein part of milk is used to make cheese. The fat part is used to make butter.

Some individuals handle dairy fairly well. Many do not. They might have an allergy to the milk protein, or they may lack the enzyme to digest the lactose. In fact, about 70% of humans are lactose intolerant to a certain degree.

For those who do not handle cow's milk well, goat's milk might be an excellent alternative. Here are some advantages of goat's milk:
- In general, goat's milk is more like human milk than cow's milk.
- Goat's milk is digested much more quickly than cow's milk.
- Because the protein of goat's milk is more easily digested, it is less likely to produce allergic reactions and is less mucus forming.
- It has less lactose and is therefore less likely to cause bloating and gas.
- The fat in goat's milk is more easily digested and includes a higher proportion of medium chain fatty acids that benefit the immune system and inhibit the growth of yeast.
- Compared to cow's milk, goat's milk has higher levels of calcium, vitamin B-6, potassium, niacin, and selenium.

Raw Milk

Government agencies warn of the dangers of raw milk, while assuring us that pasteurized milk is safe, and of excellent food value.[4] However, traditional farmers claim that if you feed pasteurized milk to a calf, it will likely die in about six weeks.

Pasteurization oxidizes the milk fat, while altering the protein so that it is more difficult to digest. Pasteurization destroys the enzymes that allow us to utilize the nutrients. Heat makes the calcium in milk less compatible for the body, causing it to form arterial deposits.

Raw milk is significantly more nutritious and easier to utilize than pasteurized milk. However, it is illegal to sell raw milk for human consumption in most states in the United Sates. You can often buy raw goat or cow milk directly from certain farmers, if you explain that you are getting it for your cat.

If you do want to drink the pasteurized milk, buy organic milk, especially organic goat's milk, and use it in moderation. Pay attention to your body signals. Any adverse reactions, such as gas, diarrhea, constipation, or congestion, are signs that you should reduce consumption, or eliminate it entirely.

Fermented Foods

Fermentation is a process by which food is partially broken down by bacteria or fungi, producing a wealth of beneficial byproducts, such as vitamins, amino acids, lactic acid, and enzymes. Fermented foods are an excellent way of getting some of the nutrients that may be deficient in the diet, due to the lack of fresh and raw foods. Fermentation also increases the digestibility of foods that otherwise might be problematic, such as dairy and soy.

Many traditional diets around the world use fermented foods, especially in the cooler climates, where fresh fruits and vegetables are less available. Two of the diets described in chapter 9, the Macrobiotic Diet and Weston A. Price Diet, make liberal use of fermented foods.

When buying fermented foods, read the label to make sure the product really is fermented, and really does contain a significant amount of live cultures and their byproducts. Better yet, make the fermented products at home.

Examples of Fermented Foods

- **Sauerkraut:** Fermented cabbage.
- **Pickles:** Fermented cucumbers.
- **Miso, tempeh, natto, soy sauce:** Fermented soy products.
- **Fermented milk products:** Milk is fermented by infusing it with bacteria that convert the milk sugar (lactose) into lactic acid. The acid causes the milk protein to solidify (curdle). Depending on the bacteria that are used, the milk will initially turn into buttermilk, yogurt or kefir. If the solid curd is allowed to separate from the liquid part of the milk (whey), the curd forms cheese. Like other fermented foods, fermented milk products provide beneficial bacteria and their byproducts. Since most of the lactose has been converted into lactic acid, fermented dairy is better tolerated by individuals with lactose intolerance. Furthermore, some of the enzymes produced by the bacteria assist in digesting the milk protein and fat. Fermented milk products are especially beneficial when made from raw milk. Even in places where it is not legal to sell raw milk, raw cheese is still available.

See Appendix C for more information on fermented foods, including instructions on how to make sauerkraut.

Replacement Foods

The bottom line for healthy eating is to favor whole foods that have had minimal processing. However, for those individuals who are used to the convenience, taste, and texture of fast foods, here are some alternatives:

Soy Burgers and Soy Franks

These products are highly processed and often contain toxic substances. The toxicity issue is compounded if the products are made from commercially grown soy — which means the beans are probably GMO (in the United States, anyway).

Are store-bought soy burgers and franks better than fast-food beef burgers and hot dogs? That depends. If your primary consideration is to eat healthier, the choice between meat-based and soy-based fast foods might be a bit like the choice between fried pork skins and potato chips. Actually, the soy might win out when we consider what goes into fast-food "beef" burgers and franks. However, choosing the lesser of two evils is not the same as choosing for optimum health. The soy analogues of burgers and franks are not the sort of food you would eat regularly as "health foods."

If you enjoy soy-based burgers, make them yourself from organic tofu or tempeh. Also, for the sake of not overdoing it with the soy, make your own patties from other legumes, such as black beans and lentils — very inexpensive and quite delicious.

Non-dairy Cheese

The main choices are almond, rice, and soy cheese. These cheese-like products tend to be highly processed. If you specifically want to try them as a way of reducing your dairy, be aware that many "non-dairy" cheeses do have casein (milk protein) as one of the ingredients.

Non-dairy Ice Cream

If you really like ice cream, nothing replaces it. However, non-dairy frozen treats can offer a tasty alternative when you feel like having a dessert that resembles ice cream, in texture and sweetness, but want to avoid dairy. You can also make some surprisingly tasty, satisfying, quick and inexpensive raw "ice-cream" from blended frozen fruits, such as bananas, with perhaps some nuts and seeds for a creamier texture.

A Guide to Milk Alternatives

If you wish to reduce or eliminate dairy products, but would like to continue to enjoy the experience of consuming something that resembles milk, here are some alternatives.:

- *Soy milk* is readily available and relatively inexpensive. Since soy is a legume, the protein complements the whole grain cereal that you place it on. However, soy milk is not as nutritionally complete as dairy milk, and should not be viewed as a nutritional replacement for it. Like other unfermented soy products, soy milk is not that easy to digest and contains substances (such as phytoestrogens) that could be detrimental for some individuals, especially if consumed in large amounts. Therefore, as with dairy milk, do not depend on it as a staple food, choose organic (to avoid the GMO), and use it in moderation.

- *Rice milk* is hypoallergenic and easier to digest than soy milk. However, as with soy milk, it is still not as nutritionally complete as dairy milk. Therefore, do not rely on it as a staple, but use it when you feel like having some "milk" as a quick beverage or to put on your cereal.
- *Coconut milk.* The liquid part of the coconut, though pleasantly sweet, is generally too watery to serve as a milk substitute for most people. However, when the water from a young coconut is blended with some of the coconut meat, the two combine into a delicious and satisfying drink that, for many individuals, replaces the flavor, texture and satisfying quality of dairy milk.
- *Nut/seed milk* has a closer resemblance to dairy milk, compared to soy and rice milk. For example, it provides a significant amount of protein and is rich in beneficial fats. Nuts and seeds also tend to be rich in minerals and phytonutrients. Unlike soy, which is high in omega-6 oils, many nuts and seeds provide omega-3 oils. The most readily available nut/seed milk on the market is almond milk. However, nut/seed milk is best when it is made at home and consumed right away.

As dairy alternatives, all four of the above milk-substitutes can vary greatly in quality. Read the label. Look for organic ingredients and a minimum amount (zero, preferably) of added sugar. Also, be aware that the store-bought milk alternatives that are not refrigerated often come in cartons that are typically lined with aluminum. The cleanest, most nutritious, and inexpensive way to make nut and seed milk is to make it at home.

How to Make Nut and Seed Milk at Home

Here are the nuts and seeds that are most commonly used to make milk.
- Almonds are tasty and tend to have a higher protein and lower fat content than other nuts and seeds.
- Flax seeds are an excellent source of omega-3 fats.
- Walnuts are loaded with nutrients that benefit the brain.
- Brazil nuts are extremely rich in selenium. One Brazil nut easily provides the daily recommended allowance of selenium. For the same reason, use them sparingly.
- Pumpkin seeds are rich in zinc and have oils that help to eliminate intestinal parasites.

Here are a few simple ways to make nut and seed milk.

Using a very powerful blender:
- Blend one cup of almonds, and a tablespoon of flax seeds or chia seeds with 20-32 ounces of water. Vary the water to create the desired consistency.
- You can vary the proportion of almonds to flax/chia seeds to change the flavor or nutritional profile.
- You can remove the pulp from the blended milk by using a sieve or cheese cloth.

Using a coffee grinder and regular blender:
- Grind up the almonds and flax seeds in the coffee grinder.
- Blend the powder with enough water to make a beverage of desired consistency.

Variations:
- Sweeten with honey, maple syrup or dates.
- Use other nuts and seeds, such as walnuts, sunflower seeds, Brazil nuts, and pumpkin seeds for variety of flavor and nutritional content.
- The water may be reduced to make pudding, which can then be frozen as "ice cream."

What about Babies?

Babies and young children often have problems with cow's milk. Furthermore, there is evidence that giving young children (especially babies before age two) cow's milk can trigger type I diabetes.

Nonetheless, the above four milk alternatives are not very suitable for infants. Soy milk is of special concern, for the reasons given earlier in this chapter, as well as having high levels of glutamate, an amino acid that is known to over-stimulate and damage brain cells, when introduced in large concentrations. The most common source of glutamate is a condiment called monosodium glutamate (MSG). Also, for infants (first three months), the high levels of phytoestrogens in soy formula could disrupt sexual development. Boys tend to not know whether they are boys or girls, and girls mature very early, often reaching puberty by the age of eight![5] Mothers who are unable to breast feed their infants and would like to avoid formulas that are based on cow's milk, can explore other options, such as a wet nurse, a milk bank, or goat's milk.

Chapter 5
The Other Side of Nutrition

To find your ideal diet, bear in mind that good nutrition has two sides — feeding and cleansing. Most diets described in chapter 9 emphasize the nutrient content of food, while neglecting the toxic residue. This oversight is often the very reason many diets prove to be unsustainable in the long run.

> **Your Ideal Diet**
> Your ideal diet provides the proper balance of all needed nutrients in the cleanest and most digestible form possible.

Toxicity does not necessarily have to come from obviously toxic chemicals that have no nutritive value. Toxicity can also come from needed nutrients eaten in excessive amounts that simply overtax the body's capacity for digestion and cleanup.

Excess = Toxicity

Though an unbalanced diet is likely to have both deficiency and excess, the first sign of problems is usually toxicity, due to excess. For example, indigestion and unwanted weight gain are two common symptoms resulting from simply over-consuming calories.

The correlation between excess and toxicity is an important one, because we tend to equate "more" with "better." You might be persuaded to purchase a concentrated powdered food supplement because it has "more protein," but do you actually need the extra protein, and is it increasing the toxic burden on the body?

To complicate matters, even in the absence of overt signs of toxicity (such as nausea, fatigue, and skin eruptions), low-grade toxic build-up can still be present. It may develop so gradually as to be virtually undetectable until serious pathologies arise. For example, the first sign of cardiovascular problems is sometimes a fatal heart attack.

Though any nutrient can become toxic in large enough amounts, some nutrients reach their toxic threshold faster than others. The typical scenario is to have an excess of macronutrients (carbohydrates, fats, and protein) and a deficiency of micronutrients (vitamins, minerals, and phytonutrients. For example, the degenerative changes in arteries that eventually lead to the heart attack occur silently over a period of years, and may be traced to diets that are high in sodium, saturated fats, oxidized cholesterol, and trans-fats, with an associated deficiency of vitamin C, vitamin B_{12}, folate, and omeg -3 oils.

The Cause of Disease

On the purely physical level, all disease can be traced to toxicity or deficiency. This includes all the major degenerative diseases associated with modern living (cardiovascular disease, cancer, diabetes, arthritis, etc.), as well as rapid aging. More specifically, we eat too many calories and not enough vitamins, minerals and phytonutrients.

Furthermore, toxicity and deficiency do not act independently. They play off of each other. For example, any toxic condition is made worse by a lack of micronutrients, because one of their jobs is to help the body dispose of toxins.

Eating a clean and balanced diet becomes easier when we favor whole foods, while reducing or totally avoiding food-extracts, such as vegetable oil, butter, tofu, and cheese. Toxicity and deficiency become more likely as we consume substantial amounts of products that are not whole foods. For example, when olive oil is extracted from its whole food matrix, many nutrients are removed, while other nutrients (most notably, the oil itself) become highly concentrated and can overtax the body's capacity to process them.

Common Sources of Toxicity

The toxic effect of excessive macronutrients begins in the digestive system, simply by exceeding the body's ability to digest these nutrients, and continues when they are absorbed into the blood. Of the three macronutrients, protein is the one that gets over-consumed most frequently. Excessive protein promotes the growth of putrefactive bacteria and other parasites in the intestines. In addition, the extra amino acids are broken down by our cells, resulting in the production of ammonia and other metabolic poisons.

The toxicity of fat is primarily due to the fact that it is not water soluble, which means it can potentially "clog" the body and impede absorption of oxygen, glucose, and other nutrients by the cells. The toxicity of fats is compounded when they have been oxidized through heating, processing, and exposure to oxygen.

Carbohydrates are generally processed more quickly and easily than protein and fat. However, that advantage becomes a disadvantage when carbohydrates are refined and over-consumed, which is easy to do, especially when the body's ability to handle them has already been compromised by excessively high levels of fat. Below is a more detailed explanation of what happens when we over-consume macronutrients.

Too Much Carbohydrate

- An excess of sugar in the body provides food for yeast and other types of fungi.
- If carbohydrates flood the bloodstream in concentrations exceeding the body's ability to move the sugar into the cells, the result is excessive elevation (spiking) of the blood sugar. The body responds by producing high levels of insulin, which has been associated with cardiovascular disease, Alzheimer's disease, and rapid aging of the tissues.
- If the total ingested calories exceed the body's daily requirements, the extra carbohydrates are converted into fat, which is then transported through the blood. The result is elevation of blood triglycerides, and eventually, cholesterol. In other words, excess carbohydrate consumption will result in some of the same harmful effects as excess fat consumption!
- If the carbohydrates happen to be in the form of unnaturally high levels of fructose, as in high-fructose corn syrup, the conversion into fats is further accelerated.
- If the main source of carbohydrates is supplied by refined grains and starchy vegetables that have been cooked, heavily spiced, and mixed with fat (which is typical) the individual can easily over-consume calories, while being deficient in vitamins, minerals, and phytonutrients.
- Grains, like other seeds, tend to have enzyme inhibitors and anti-nutrients that block the proper digestion and absorption of nutrients.

Too Much Fat

- The main issue with fat is that it does not dissolve in water. Our tissues exist in a watery environment, and can essentially get "clogged" with too much fat.

- Though the role of fat as a primary cause of cardiovascular disease is questioned, excessive fat, especially cholesterol, saturated fat, and trans-fats, can contribute to plaquing of arteries, directly or indirectly, as described in chapter 9.
- High levels of fat in the blood are associated with decreased oxygenation of cells.
- Large amounts of stored body fat and high levels of fat in the blood have been associated with insulin resistance (Type II Diabetes).[1,2,3]
- Reduction of dietary carbohydrates mitigates some of the issues associated with higher levels of fat. This is the strategy used by low-carb diets. However, when the dietary carbohydrates are *very* low, the burning of fat results in higher levels of ketones, such as acetone. This is why individuals who fast, or go on a severely carbohydrate-restricted diet, often have "acetone breath." These ketones tend to acidify the blood and irritate the kidneys. In addition, elevated ketones have been associated with tumor growth.[4]
- Foods that are naturally high in fat are often (though not necessarily) also high in protein. Therefore, the above issues with fat are likely to be accompanied by toxicity from too much protein, as described below.

Too Much Protein
- If ingested protein exceeds the amount we actually need to maintain the body, the excess is simply burned for energy. However, when the cells break down amino acids, ammonia is produced. The liver converts this highly toxic chemical into urea and perhaps uric acid, which are much less toxic, though not completely harmless. In addition, the body also gets an immediate dose of these waste products upon eating the meat, because, when the animal is slaughtered, urea and uric acid and other toxic waste products begin to accumulate in the meat, even when frozen.
- If protein consumption is high enough, the amount of ammonia produced by the cells can exceed the liver's ability to detoxify it, producing nausea. To avoid this, most diets guide the individual away from eating the very high levels of protein that have been shown to precipitate such an episode.
- However, long before we reach the point of nausea from liver toxicity, the body can still be subjected to irritants and metabolic poisons from high protein foods. For example, the extra uric acid can easily form crystals

that irritate tissues, most notably joints and kidneys. If the uric acid levels are high enough, the joint irritation can result in gout, and the crystals in the kidneys can grow into painful stones. In the absence of these obvious signs, the subclinical (hidden) irritation can continue for years, contributing to the degradation and rapid aging of the kidneys and other vital organs. Here is an excerpt from an article by Owen Parrett, M.D.:

"Beefsteak contains about 14 grains of uric acid per pound. ...The uric acid accounts for the quick pickup a steak seems to give, much like a cup of coffee gives. Uric acid, or trioxypurin, closely resembles caffeine... The late Dr. L. H. Newburg, of the University of Michigan, called attention to the fact that when meat formed 25 percent of a rat's diet, the rat became bigger and more active than rats on a normal diet. But after a few months, the kidneys of the meat-eating rat became badly damaged."[5]

Figure 5.1: The Toxicity Scale

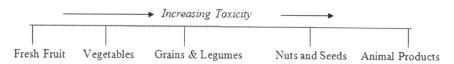

The "scale" in figure 5.1 is not really a scale, for the obvious reason that it has no numbers. It is not intended to be a precise representation of toxicity in any given food (which would be difficult to quantify), but rather to help us visualize the *relative* toxicity of the various food groups. Animal products, nuts, seeds, and grains require more digestive effort and cleanup than fruits and low-starch vegetables. Likewise, a pound of strawberries requires less digestion and cleanup than a pound of kale.

The difference in toxicity is partially due to cooking, which seems to destroy nutrients and produce toxins, as suggested by two early studies in the 1930s and 40s.[6,7] Unfortunately, follow-up studies have not been done on either one of these, so they have remained unconfirmed. However, subsequent research has shown that cooking does, indeed, produce certain toxic chemicals. For example:
- Cooking carbohydrates produces carcinogenic substances called acrylomides.[8]
- Cooking oxidizes fats, making them toxic.[9]
- Cooking protein produces protein-carbohydrate complexes that promote low-grade inflammation, degeneration, and aging of tissues.[10]

Higher temperatures and longer cooking time results in higher toxicity. However, with some foods, cooking can *decrease* toxicity. For example, some vegetables contain low-grade irritants that are partially or totally neutralized by cooking. In the case of beans, soaking and cooking removes or neutralizes toxic compounds. In the case of animal products and some plant foods, cooking also serves the purpose of destroying pathogens.

Another factor that influences the toxic burden of any food is the number of calories provided by the meal. For example, compared to a pound of romaine lettuce, one pound of cooked grains and legumes requires more digestion and cleanup, because the latter two pack more calories. For similar reasons, nuts and seeds require even more digestion and cleanup. For example, a meal featuring a pound of cooked rice and lentils provides about 550 calories. In contrast, one pound of walnuts packs almost 3000 calories. Eating that many nuts and seeds in one sitting constitutes "binging" for most individuals. The body quickly lets you know it would prefer you not do that on a regular basis. In addition to providing more calories, nuts and seeds are also very high in fat and can therefore stress the liver if consumed in large amounts, especially when roasted and salted.

Animal products typically have lower total fat than nuts and seeds, but are much higher in protein, saturated fat, and cholesterol, all three of which are usually subjected to high cooking temperatures and oxidation, thus increasing their toxic effects on the body. However, with animal products, the harmful effects tend to accumulate gradually and silently. Therefore, the same individual who would not think of eating a pound of nuts and seeds, might eat one or two pounds of cooked meat, eggs, and dairy on a daily basis. and think nothing of it.

The above description of the relative toxicity of the various food groups should not be taken to mean that animal products, grains, nuts, and seeds are bad, while fruits and vegetables are good. The idea is to have the right proportion of the various food groups to allow for proper nourishment and cleansing.

Building-foods and Cleansing-foods

Grains, legumes, nuts, seeds, and animal products have been called "building-foods" because they provide the concentrated calories and building material to grow and maintain the body. On the other hand, fruits and low-starch vegetables have been called "cleansing-foods" because they are lower in calories, while providing an abundance of vitamins, alkalizing minerals, antioxidants, water, and plant fiber, all of which are important for cleansing and detoxification.

In other words, the same high concentration of macronutrients that makes some foods taxing and potentially toxic also makes them valuable for building and maintaining the body. For example, on the extreme right hand side of the above toxicity scale, animal products have, by far, the highest levels of protein, which makes them powerful building-foods for promoting regeneration. However, that same feature also makes them toxic if over-consumed on a regular basis.

The good news is that the high concentration of protein and other nutrients found in animal products also means we do not have to consume very large quantities in order to obtain significant levels of these nutrients. The same applies to nuts, seeds, and to a lesser extent, grains and legumes. In general, the more calorically-dense the food, the less we need to consume to receive its benefits. Naturally, the ideal proportion of building-foods and cleansing-foods can vary from person to person, and can even change for the same individual over time. The body's requirements can fluctuate with the seasons, climate, and the level of physical and emotional stress.

But What Should I Eat?

Ultimately, this question must be answered by the individual seeking the answer. However, the general guidelines given in chapter 1 still apply and may be summarized as follows: *Fulfill as much of your nutritional requirements as you can with foods that demand the least amount of digestion and cleanup.* This does not necessarily mean you should eat enormous amounts of fruits and vegetables and very little of everything else. This is where instinct is important. The principle of selecting the cleanest foods possible is useful, but does not replace your own food instincts. Your inner signals are your best guide for determining the proportion of building-foods and cleansing-foods that is right for you. The same inner signals will also guide you as to when to adjust those proportions to suit your changing needs. Chapter 11 explores the instinctual aspects of eating in more detail.

Giving the Body a Rest

Eating habits that trigger physical degeneration invariably subject the body to excessive amounts of the building-foods and not enough of the cleansing-foods – too many calories and not enough vitamins, minerals, and phytonutrients. Likewise, the general strategy for any "cleansing program" is to temporarily reduce the building-foods and increase the cleansing-foods. This way, the body can catch up on the backlog of accumulated debris. This is accomplished by simply decreasing the animal products, grains, legumes, nuts, and seeds, while increasing fruits and vegetables.

Yes, it is that simple. However, simple is not the same as easy. We can more effectively implement this simple strategy if we first take the time to fully understand why some foods generate more toxicity than others. To do so, let us first consider the process of digestion.

Digestion

The nutritional value and potential toxicity of any food is greatly influenced by the body's ability to digest it properly. Digestion is the process of dissolving food so as to extract the nutrients needed by the body.

After food is swallowed, it sits in the stomach for a while, then progresses to the small intestine, and then the large intestine. During this journey, the nutrients are extracted from the food and are absorbed into the blood. However, to the extent that digestion and absorption are compromised, the nutrients lingering in the digestive tract provide food for bacteria and other microbes. Some of the bacteria actually produce beneficial substances, but others produce toxins, including some potent carcinogens (cancer-causing substances). These inwardly-produced toxins add to the burden produced by chemicals already present in the food.

The way to protect the body from toxicity is to select the cleanest foods possible, while occasionally giving special attention to body cleansing.

Cleansing the Large Intestine

Due to the presence of microorganisms, the large intestine tends to be the dirtiest place in the body. The toxins from the large intestine are absorbed into the blood and taken straight to the liver, which detoxifies them as best as it can. Toxins that the liver is not able to adequately break down and eliminate go back into the blood and must be expelled though the kidneys, lungs, and skin. Therefore, whatever we can do to reduce the burden on these organs of elimination can ultimately have a profound effect on our health.

The general guideline for maintaining a clean large intestine is to have a bowel movement at least once a day (preferably more). However, due to years of stress, many individuals' transit time is 2-3 days or longer. The resultant toxicity is believed to contribute to a wide variety of degenerative conditions, including cancer and arthritis.

During its extended sojourn in the large intestine, the food-residue provides a fertile breeding ground for putrefactive bacteria and other microbes whose toxic byproducts continuously seep into the blood and bathe the cells of the body. In addition, some of the residue can become caked onto the wall of the large intestine, allowing larger parasites (worms) to proliferate.

The most obvious indicator of the large intestine's level of hygiene is the smell of the feces during a bowel movement. Of course, it will not smell like roses, but neither should it make roses wither away. The offensive or noxious odor is Mother Nature's signal that toxic chemicals are present. The simplest, safest, cheapest, and most natural way to cleanse the large intestine is to just allow it to cleanse itself, by increasing the amount of fresh and raw fruits and vegetables, rich in fiber and water. Meanwhile, the heavier foods, especially those very rich in fat and protein, are reduced or avoided for a while.

Cleansing the Liver

Nutrients and toxins that enter the blood from the intestines go straight to the liver. After the large intestine has been allowed to cleanse itself, the individual can simply continue to eat an abundance of raw fruits and vegetables, while perhaps taking additional steps to promote additional liver cleansing:

- Increase dark green leafy vegetables, such as fresh dandelion, spinach, and kale.
- Increase cruciferous vegetables such as kale, broccoli, and Brussels sprouts.
- Drink apple juice. Use organic apple juice because conventionally grown apples are usually sprayed heavily.
- Drink carrot juice and beet juice — about 6 parts carrot to 1 part beet. Limit the overall dose to 10 ounces or so — or less, if the person has blood sugar issues.
- Drink lemon juice: ½-1 lemon in warm water every morning.

Cleansing the Kidneys

The kidneys are filters that remove waste from the blood. In that regard, they are similar to the liver. However, the liver has the capacity to remove large molecules that do not dissolve well in water, whereas the kidneys remove small, water-soluble molecules. In other words, as a filter, the kidney is finer and more delicate than the liver, and is more easily damaged by physical or chemical irritants. The simplest and safest way to keep the kidneys clean is to drink ample amounts of clean water, while increasing the amount of juicy fruits in diet, such as watermelon and cucumbers. Individuals who have kidneys issues are also advised to be moderate with ingested protein.

Cleansing the Lungs and Skin

Deep breathing and exercise are easy ways of to cleanse the lungs and skin. Elimination through the skin is more important than most individuals realize. One pound of waste may be discharged though the skin every day. Here are some ways to promote skin cleansing:
- Dry skin brushing. Use a loofa, coarse brush, or rough towel.
- Hot (3 minutes) and cold (30 seconds) showers to stimulate circulation through the skin (not for individuals who have a heart condition).
- Induce sweating through exercise or sauna.

Body Cleansing and Exercise

Exercise promotes cleansing of *all* portals of elimination, as well as promoting good digestion, enhancing the immune system, elevating emotions, reducing food cravings, and stabilizing blood sugar and blood pressure. The health improvement through diet change can be limited by a sedentary lifestyle. This might be the reason a given diet "doesn't work" for a given individual. In other words, the person was seeking a dietary solution to a problem stemming from a lack of exercise. Exercise allows *any* given diet to work better! Not surprisingly, virtually all the dietary systems promote exercise.

Clean Body and Clear Mind

The almost immediate psychological benefits of exercise are testimony to the powerful connection between physical and psychological health. That connection includes a need for physical cleansing as a prerequisite for a properly functioning mind. In particular, a clean and well-functioning digestive system seems to be essential for mental clarity and emotional serenity. A toxic and constipated large intestine will contribute to "poopy thoughts." The mere fact that psychological health is called "sanity" reminds us of its intimate connection to "sanitation."

The One-day Cleanse

This cleanse can be done for one or more days. If you find it is beneficial, you can do it once a week, every other week, or once a month. This process is especially effective if you also exercise outdoors during the day, especially in the morning before breakfast.

Morning

After your brisk morning exercise, you can use any of the following options for breakfast:

- Just drink water until lunch time (unless you have blood sugar issues).
- Freshly squeezed vegetable juice.
- A mono-fruit meal consisting of one type of fresh fruit.
- A smoothie made of green leafy vegetables and enough fresh fruit to make it tasty.

Afternoon

- A green smoothie.
- A fruit mono-meal.
- A raw vegetable salad. Use a low-fat dressing consisting of any combination of the following: lemon juice, orange juice, blended tomato, mango or strawberries, chunks of soaked sun-dried tomatoes, raw or lightly cooked mushrooms.
- Fruit followed by a vegetable salad.
- If you get hungry between lunch and dinner, have fresh fruit or a green smoothie.

Evening

- For dinner, you can use the same basic options as lunch, perhaps with a different combination of ingredients.
- The same fruits and vegetables used to make the salad dressing can also be rearranged into a delicious raw soup, which can replace or complement the salad.
- If you get hungry after dinner, you can have a fruit snack.

Chapter 6
Guidelines for Healthy Eating

Ideally, good nutrition should be as simple as eating whatever appeals to you, but many individuals find it challenging. To understand why, let us consider animals in the wild. The nervous system of wild animals is designed to monitor and regulate raw and unprocessed whole foods, usually one item at a time. The human nervous system is fundamentally the same. It is designed to track raw food, one item at time. Under these conditions, whatever tastes good is also good for you. The brain can easily discern when you have eaten enough, at which point you feel satisfied and therefore stop eating.

On the other hand, the cooking, refining, and mixing of foods exposes us to chemicals and combinations of chemicals that our nervous system is not designed to handle. Consequently, the food may taste and smell good, but is not necessarily beneficial. For example, in the wild, a whole food that tastes sweet, such as fruit, contains nutrients in concentrations and proportions we can easily handle. However, if we extract the sugar from that fruit and use it to sweeten things that are normally bad-tasting or bland, such as partially hydrogenated vegetable oil and refined wheat flour (as in commercially produced cookies and cakes), we trick our nervous system; we feel pleasure even though we are consuming large amounts of food that is nutritionally unbalanced and leaves a substantial toxic residue.

This does not mean we should totally abstain from all food except for raw, unprocessed, and unmixed. The point is this: to the extent we eat food in a manner other than how nature presents it, our eating instincts will have a harder time guiding us. Therefore, for most individuals, healthy food choice is a combination of two things:
- Instinct (taste and intuition)
- Educated common sense.

The educated part of common sense is the study of nutrition, which can get rather complicated. However, we do have some simple guidelines, as described below.

> ## General Guidelines for Healthy Eating
> - Get as much of your nutrition as you can from foods that require the least digestion and have the lowest toxic residue — fruits and low-starch vegetables. As we increase our fresh fruits and vegetables, eating becomes progressively simpler.
> - Add the appropriate amount of the heavier foods as needed — legumes, nuts, seeds, and animal products.
> - For better digestion, avoid eating food that is too hot or too cold. Very hot foods debilitate the stomach, and very cold foods take vitality from the system, inhibiting digestion.
> - Minimize or eliminate fluids with meals. Ideally, do not drink for one-half hour before the meal, and for one hour after.
> - If you tend to feel "stuffed" after you eat, eat more slowly so your brain has a chance to catch up with your stomach. Another trick is to stop eating when you feel about 80% full — which is easier to accomplish if you eat slowly. In fact, if you just put your attention on eating more slowly, you might find that you automatically eat about 20% less. In other words, you eat until you are satisfied, but you give your brain more time to realize that the stomach is full.
> - Eat your last meal of the day 2-3 hours before you go to bed. The stomach needs to rest and regenerate at night.
> - For better digestion, you can practice proper food combining.
> - Chew your food thoroughly. In addition to physically breaking down the food for better digestion, chewing stimulates secretion of digestive juices further on down.

Food Combining

In the natural world, foods that are high in fat also tend to be high in protein, and proportionately lower in carbohydrates. For example, beef provides all of its calories in the form of fat and protein, having virtually no carbohydrates. On the other hand, fruits, vegetables, legumes, and grains tend to provide most of the calories from carbohydrates with relatively small contributions from fat and protein. Grains and legumes do have a nutritionally significant amount of protein, but carbohydrates still dominate.

The combination that typically does not occur in our naturally occurring foods is one featuring a high level of both carbohydrates *and* fats.

Nonetheless, that combination is very common in our own culinary creations: cookies, cakes, ice-cream, pizza, ham sandwiches with mayo, potato chips, French fries, etc. Here are the main issues arising with this combination:

- **Overeating.** When a meal has both concentrated fats and concentrated carbohydrates, it is easy to over-consume calories. In such a situation, the body will preferentially burn the carbohydrates and store the fats — because that is what the body is designed to do. *This is a major contributor to unwanted weight gain.*
- **Digestive disturbance.** Carbohydrates digest relatively fast, while fats and proteins require more time. It is, therefore, not surprising that digestion is best when we do not mix large amounts of high-carb food with large amounts of high-fat and protein foods. When the three are all mixed in large amounts, the fat and protein slow down the digestion of carbohydrates, which, in turn, provide food for gas-producing bacteria and yeast.
- **Blood sugar issues.** High levels of fat in the blood slow down the passage of blood sugar into the cells. Therefore, a diet featuring high levels of both fat and carbohydrates is more likely to gradually lead to insulin resistance and diabetes mellitus. This is especially true with a diet that features the wrong kind of fats combined with refined carbohydrates — as in the typical processed foods.

The general principle for proper food combining is to avoid mixing foods that differ widely with regard to time spent in the stomach. Food requiring a short transit time, such as fruit, will be "stalled" in the stomach and rot if it has to wait on another food that has a longer transit time, such as meat, dairy, or fatty plant foods. Therefore, the rule of thumb for food combining is to keep high protein/fat foods separate from high carbohydrate foods. Based on this principle, proper food combining can be summarized as the following four guidelines:

- Low-starch vegetables combine well with animal products, nuts and seeds, starchy vegetables, and grains.
- Eat fruits separate from other foods.
- Eat melons separate from other fruits.
- Acid fruits, such as oranges, do not combine well with sweet fruits, such as bananas. Acid fruits combine fairly well with subacid (apples). Subacids combine fairly well with sweet fruit.

How Important Is Food Combining?

Most individuals would probably benefit from not mixing large amounts of fruits with other foods that require an extended sojourn in the stomach. Beyond that, food combining may or may not be necessary for a given individual. In general, the more sensitive or "slow" your digestive system, the more likely that you would benefit from practicing food combining. For example, some individuals seem to experience no obvious digestive issues with tofu and rice (protein and carbs), or a fish sandwich with mayo (protein, fat, and carbs). However the absence of obvious gastric disturbance does not necessarily mean that all is well with the rest of the body. As mentioned above, the simultaneous presence of high levels of fats and carbohydrates in the diet (especially the wrong kind of both) could gradually lead to blood sugar issues.

For more information on food combining, see Appendix A.

Food Preparation

There are two major options for food preparation: cooked or raw.

Suggestions for raw food preparation:

- Soak or sprout nuts and seeds. (Note: limit the sprouting process to the very early stages. Soaking is adequate to soften the seeds and neutralize some of the irritants and antinutrients. Sprouting can increase these benefits, but can also create other problems if allowed to progress too far.
- In addition to just cutting up vegetables and making a salad, you can shred or grind them for easier chewing and variety of flavor and texture.
- Vegetables that are relatively soft and fleshy, such as zucchini, yellow squash, and cucumbers can be quickly shredded. You can then throw them on a salad or serve as a side dish, seasoned to your taste.
- Using a simple gadget called the spiral slicer; you can turn various vegetables into something that looks like spaghetti. Zucchini spaghetti has its own subtle flavor and texture, which you can then embellish with the topping of your choice, including raw or cooked tomato sauce.
- Coarser vegetables such as carrots, celery, and beets can be finely ground with a grater or other simple kitchen tools. Finely ground carrots have a delightful flavor and texture.
- Rediscover the natural flavor of unprocessed foods. Experiment with very simple meals such as a fruit mono-meal.

Suggestions for cooked food preparation

One of the best investments you can make for promoting long-term health is to replace aluminum and Teflon cookware with stainless steel, porcelain, or glass. The aluminum does get into the food. The longer you cook the food, the higher the aluminum content. This is especially true with acidic foods that naturally react with metals, such as tomato sauce. If you cook a tomato-rich meal in an aluminum container and then let it sit for several hours, it can absorb dangerous levels of aluminum. Individuals who eat such leftovers can get so ill they have to be rushed to the hospital.[68] However, even if you do not allow such extremely high levels of aluminum to accumulate, the low levels that are added every time you use aluminum cookware or eat leftovers wrapped in aluminum foil can still accumulate in the body over time — especially the brain.

What is wrong with Teflon? Small pets, such as birds, have died from the fumes that are emitted from Teflon cookware. Furthermore, the manufacturing of Teflon releases the same chemical (perfluorooctanoic acid or PFRA), which has been found in wells far removed from the factory. That chemical has been linked to various ailments in animals, including cancer, liver damage, birth defects, and immune system suppression. It has also been linked to birth defects and other ailments in humans. In addition, such chemicals (fluorinated hydrocarbons) interfere with the brains ability to think clearly. Every time you cook with Teflon cookware, PFRA gets into the food you eat and the air you breathe.

Organically Grown

The body attains optimum health to the extent that we allow it to harmonize with the cycles and rhythms of nature. The body degenerates when we do not allow it to do so. Ultimately, what we do to the environment, we do to ourselves, because we are part of the cycles of nature. When we eat artificial foods and dump toxic chemicals into the environment, we disrupt the cycles and rhythms of nature and degrade our food supply. The results are predictable.

One way to harmonize with nature is to eat organically grown whole foods. According to the current federal organic standards, food is considered organically grown if it is grown without insecticides, herbicides, antibiotics, or other synthetic chemicals, and free of genetic engineering. The term organically grown also implies the soil itself is kept in good condition. However, FDA currently permits small amounts of pesticides to be used with certain crops and allows them to still be labeled as Certified Organic. Private organic certifying standards tend to be stricter in this regard.

Reasons for Buying Organic

- Organically grown food tends to be higher in minerals.[1]
- Organic farming preserves the soil organisms that produce vitamins, such as B_{12}.
- Organic food tastes better.
- Most of the conventionally grown foods have detectable levels of pesticides, while most of the organically grown foods do not. 60% of all herbicides, 90% of all fungicides, and 30% of all insecticides are potentially carcinogenic.
- When farmers use herbicides and pesticides, they are infusing our food with chemicals that are designed to kill living things. Pesticides are specifically designed to destroy the nervous system — they are essentially the same chemicals (such as "nerve gas") that were used in chemical warfare. To assume they will do no harm to us when routinely sprayed on food defies all common sense, and is, in fact, contrary to the data that been collected since we started using these chemicals. For example: Conventional farmers have the highest rates of certain cancers, as do their children. Other studies suggest a link between pesticides and birth defects in areas close to agricultural fields. Still other studies suggest that women who grew up in agricultural areas are more likely to have children with birth defects.[2] Field workers growing non-organic strawberries are required to wear hazmat suits while spraying the crops, because of the toxicity of the chemical that they utilize, which leaves a toxic residue in the fruit.
- Organic farming protects topsoil. Conventional farming erodes topsoil. The soil that does remain is continuously depleted of minerals. Organic farming builds soil. Organic farming maintains a rich supply of humus in the soil, which holds water, thus protecting the soil from drought, flooding, and erosion.
- Organic farming maintains "living" soil by supporting the soil food web, which includes symbiotic relationships between the plants and soil organisms.
- Organic farming helps to maintain genetic diversity. In contrast, modern farming practices and GMO crops reduce diversity and foster a monoculture, which increase the likelihood of massive crop failures.
- Why are these blatantly unhealthy practices allowed to continue? The simple answer is that we, the people, allow it.

Part II
THE DIETS

The Diets of our Ancestors

How to Evaluate any Diet

Survey of Major Diets

Okay, Let's Eat

CHAPTER 7
The Diets of Our Ancestors

How important is this chapter? That depends on the reader. If you have no interest in learning about the diets of our ancestors, but simply want to find *your* ideal diet, you can probably just skip to the next chapter. The historical and pre-historical perspective offered here is useful only if you wish to have a deeper understanding of the various diets, by considering each one against a background of what might be considered our ancestral or "natural" food.

What *Is* Our Natural Food?

The various dietary systems described in chapter 9 often use historical and pre-historical data to validate their teachings, each one claiming to possess the natural diet for humans. How is it possible for divergent nutritional theories to use essentially the same body of knowledge to support their respective ideas? Quite simply, this particular body of knowledge is vast, with much room for creative interpretation. Dietary authors might key in on a specific culture and/or period in human history or pre-history that happens to support a given dietary theory, while ignoring evidence to the contrary. The reader, not having studied human origins, can become confused.

Therefore, this chapter presents a picture of human origins that takes into account all available data that I found to be relevant to the subject of healthy eating. By considering the bigger picture, the reader can avoid being confused by one dietary system claiming that humans are natural vegetarians, while others assure us we need to eat a substantial amount of animal products.

The good news is that the information is not as complicated as you might think. Granted, the subject of evolution is complex, however, there is an underlying simplicity. What's more, the simplifying element happens to be the very subject of this book — food!

The anatomy and physiology of any animal reflects its evolutionally history, which is driven primarily by food. Therefore, a simple way to get a clue about our own ancestral or "natural" diet is to just look at how the human body is constructed and how it works.

However, once we make our observations, we should be cautious about using such data to make hasty assumptions as to what is the optimal diet for us modern humans. This is where it can get complicated. This is where the road forks between good science and bad science. In other words, having solid data is not enough. In order for information to be really meaningful, it must be examined through the clear lens of good science.

Candor + Caution = Good Science

Good science is objective. Bad science is obscured by bias and private agenda. When we drift into bad science, we seem to ask questions, but secretly assume that we already know the answer. We seem to be seeking truth, but are actually defending our beliefs.

Lack of objectivity is a major stumbling block in the study of nutrition, resulting in a lot of arguing among its teachers, and confusion in the health-seeking public. The good news is that such objectivity is a simple skill we can all practice. Objectivity does not require formal scientific training, but rather the simple willingness to be honest with the information that is before us. As we hone our objectivity skills by just practicing honesty, we sharpen our ability to distinguish good science from bad science. The old cliché, "You can't fool an honest man," applies here.

Objectivity means we consider *all* the pertinent information, rather than conveniently ignoring things that don't support our favored theories and beliefs. For example, any reference to ancestral diets, as justification for our current food choices, should be done with caution, because the foods we eat today are very different from those of our ancestors in historic and prehistoric times. It is fine to propose a theory about the diet of our ancestors, but that does not necessarily mean that such a diet is practical for all modern humans who depend on modern food sources.

Good Science Is Like Buddhism

Objectivity means we refrain from jumping to conclusions or settling into a jaded complacency wherein we assume to know all there is to know about a given subject. In this case, we do not assume to know all there is to know about human evolution and healthy eating. The good scientist does not cling to or reject any theory that has not been positively proven or disproven. In that regard, good science resembles Buddhism. As with the Buddhist master, the good scientist responds to all beliefs and unverified theories with an uncommitted and subdued "Maybe."

The quiet neutrality of good science, like the "middle way" of Buddhism, promotes objectivity and calmness, which are especially important when considering topics such as diet or human origins — both of which tend to carry a strong emotional charge. Either one of these topics can trigger heated debate, but if we combine the two (as dietary teachers often do), strong emotional reactions are even more probable, and the quiet voice of reason can easily be drowned out.

Even scientists can be blinded by the need to believe in the infallibility or supremacy of science. On the other hand, the good scientist knows that science is at its best when we remember its limitations. The most astute evolutionary biologist is the one who remembers that the theory of evolution is, after all, a theory, subject to revision. The evidence to support the overall theory of evolution is quite compelling, but we still don't know all the hidden forces driving it.

Objectivity, as applied to nutrition, means that our primary loyalty is to the truth, not to any particular established dietary doctrine. Objectivity, as applied to the study of human origins, means we would not unquestioningly accept the creation-stories and myths of various cultures and religions, but neither would we categorically dismiss them, for they could very well hold clues about our origins — including the diets of our ancestors.

Beginning the Search

Up until recently, and for several thousand years, most humans lived on whole foods, locally produced on mineral-rich soil. It is, therefore, not surprising that some dietary systems discussed in the chapter 9, such as the Weston A. Price Diet, endeavor to promote healthy eating by advocating fresh, organic, locally grown traditional farm foods.

Looking further back, however, we see that some of these foods, such as dairy, represent recent additions to the human diet, which begs the question, how suited are we to consume them? To answer this question, we must go back beyond a few centuries, or even a few millennia. We have to go well past 10,000 years ago, before our ancestors plowed the first field and domesticated animals. We have to consider the estimated two million years in which our ancestors are believed to have been hunter/gatherers. This is precisely what the Paleolithic Diet recommends. According to this diet, we are best adapted to eat meat, fruits, and vegetables, because our Paleolithic ancestors supposedly ate these foods far longer than cultivated grains, beans, and dairy.

The potential flaw with the Paleolithic Diet is that it might not be "paleo" enough. In other words, it does not look far enough back. To fully understand the validity and potential flaws of this diet strategy, we have to look more deeply into our prehistory, back to the days of the earliest members of the human family, and then further back to the apes and monkeys inhabiting the tropical forests of Africa, some 30 million years ago. In fact, to get the most complete evolutionary picture of human nutrition, we should go back some 65 million years, for this is the immense span of time that allows for the establishment of the foundational features of the human body.

So, hold on to your hypothetical time-machine, as we journey back to that ancient world, and then sit back and watch the gradual metamorphosis that eventually culminates with us — fully modern humans, eating our modern diets, which trigger our modern diseases.

New World Order

Planet Earth, 65 million years ago: The landscape is green, and superficially resembles the forests and meadows of today. However, closer examination shows some important differences. Fruit trees are relatively new and, therefore, not nearly as diversified as today. Not surprisingly, we see none of the familiar fruit-eating animals of today.

Animal life is abundant, but nowhere do we see any evidence of humanity. In fact, we do not see any animal that even vaguely resembles humans. Our closest ancestors are small and unassuming rat-like mammals that eat insects and other such tiny things. These little fur-balls are far from being the rulers of their world. In fact, we might not even catch sight them, because they prefer to scurry about at night, lurking in the shadows, burrowing through the ground, trying not to get stepped on or eaten by the massive reptiles strutting about.

However, fate steps in to save these shy little creatures from obscurity. This time period (the late Cretaceous) also marks the demise of the dinosaurs, and the end of more than 200 million years of reptilian rule. Thus, the small mammals of the day finally have their opportunity to shine.

Happily for them, this time period also marks the beginning of millions of years of a mostly warm and wet climate that favors tropical and subtropical forests. Over time, mammals populate every continent and island on the planet. A time-lapse movie of the 30 million years that follow the demise of the dinosaurs shows mammals morphing into a dazing array of shapes and sizes, including huge herbivores three times bigger than modern elephants, and ferocious carnivores that would have laughed at the big cats of today.

Birth of the Primates – and the Primate Diet

Food is a major factor driving the evolution of animals. In this case, the mammalian diaspora was aided by the other new kid on the block – the fruit tree. The presence of fruit created a niche for any animal that could utilize it. Those insect-eating mammals fit the bill. Their small size and sharp claws made them natural tree climbers. Through time, they ate fewer insects, and more fruit, while becoming better adapted for life in the trees.

A time-lapse movie of the evolving fruit-eaters shows them growing in size, their forelimbs transforming into highly mobile arms, and their front paws spreading out into grasping hands, with five nimble fingers. Their long and sharp claws recede and flatten out into modest nails, while the outer-most finger drifts away from the other four, positioning itself to become the ancestor of the fully opposable thumb.

The head also changes. The elongated snout recedes, and the face transfigures. The dagger-like teeth give way to grinding molars. The mouth reduces in size and becomes surrounded by fleshy cheeks, as the lips become more pliable and animated. As the face flattens out, the eyes rotate to the front of the face, giving them stereoscopic vision, perfect for navigating through the trees.

In other words, over time, their appearance became progressively more human-like. The resemblance was not merely superficial. They developed color vision, especially green and red, allowing them to detect brightly colored fruit against the green leaves and blue sky. The grasping hands and nimble fingers proved to be useful for other tasks besides climbing trees and picking fruit. They were perfect for caring for the young and expressing affection, both of which were probably necessitated by what is perhaps the most striking feature of the evolving fruit eater — the brain.

The body was growing fast, but the brain was growing even faster. As the face became flatter and the mouth smaller, the top of the head rapidly expanded into a prominent dome. The evolving creatures became smarter, more emotional, affectionate, playful, and inquisitive. Eventually, these former insectivores morphed into an entirely new order of mammals, which we now call primates. They quickly rose to dominance, and to this day, rule the canopies of the tropical forests of the world.

What is the relevance of all this to our own current dietary needs? The relevance is that our fundamental body-plan (the primate body-plan) evolved as an adaptation to a diet that is calorically dominated by fruit. According to paleontologists, the first recognizable primates appeared about 60 million years ago, which means that our fruit-eating heritage goes way back.

Science and Religion Converge

Interestingly enough, when we examine our ancestors' diets from a biblical standpoint, we get an overall picture that bears a haunting resemblance to the one provided by the study of evolution. For example, what does the Bible have to say about our ancestral diet? According to Genesis 1:29, our original (presumably, perfect) diet consisted of fruits, vegetables, and their seeds. After Adam and Eve got booted out of the garden, they and their descendants had to learn to eat cooked grains, starchy vegetables, animal flesh, eggs, and milk products. Other ancient writings, such as Plato's dialogues and the Hindu scriptures, make similar assertions.

However, to properly understand this big picture, and avoid making assumptions about the "perfect diet" for modern humans, we should again remember that our foods today are different from those of antiquity. Therefore, let us refrain from jumping to conclusions, but rather look more deeply, using a lens that has been made clear by the objectivity of the scientist and the mindfulness of the Buddhist.

A Marriage Made in Heaven

For about 60 million years, fruit eating has become increasingly dominant in the primate lineage, reflecting an increasingly intimate relationship between fruit trees and fruit eaters. The success of one brought success to the other, therefore, each side rapidly evolved to better serve the other.

Cooperation is a powerful survival strategy because it allows the participants to do something that is essential for all living organisms — gather energy. Life is about energy. Food provides energy, and is therefore a major driving force in the evolution of animals. However, getting energy is only half the picture. The other half is the ability to *conserve* energy.

A major expenditure of energy for most animals and plants comes from the need to attack or defend. The simplest way to minimize this huge expense is to utilize food that is freely given. Furthermore, if the same food-source also provides safety from predators and shelter from the elements, the energy savings are enormous!

Such is the relationship between fruit-eating primates and the fruit trees. The tree simultaneously provides a safe home and abundant food supply for the primates. Meanwhile, the primates provide the tree with a cheap and simple way of spreading seeds. The fruit passes quickly through the digestive system of the primate. When the seeds are eventually "planted," they don't need a lot of stored nutrients, because the ground has already been fertilized!

Food that is so easily obtainable, digested, and absorbed, allowed the primate to conserve a great deal of energy. They grew big and strong — which means they became more effective at spreading the seeds of the fruit trees. This is how the tropics became filled with numerous lively primates and their favorite fruit trees. Both were blessed by their "choice" to make love instead of war.

Through time, the primates of the ancient world became increasingly specialized to eat fruit. They evolved into the animals we now recognize as monkeys. Some of them became larger still, lost their tails, and developed an even bigger brain. They became anthropoid (human-like) apes.

Fruitarians, but Not Strict Vegans

Contrary to the claims of some vegetarian authors, there is an old and well-established precedence for flesh eating in the primate lineage. Such precedence dates back to the insectivore ancestors. Granted, that was 65 million years ago, and if primates had stopped eating insects altogether, all vestiges of flesh-eating would have vanished. However, though their teeth, digestive system, and overall anatomy clearly became specialized to eat fruit, they apparently did retain the ability to process small amounts of animal food.

Eating insects not only gives primates the nutrients that might be in short supply in fruit, but also allows them to provide yet another service for the fruit tree — pest control. The tree doesn't have to expend as much energy trying to keep up with countless miniscule marauders. Instead, it can invest even more energy to make fruits bigger, more nutritious, and more abundant, thus allowing for an increase in the size, vitality, and numbers of the fruit-eating, insect-eliminating, and seed-spreading anthropoids. Furthermore, the additional nitrogen in the diet of primates makes their droppings that much more effective for fertilizing the ground around the tree.

In other words, the evolutionarily basis for humans eating animal flesh actually goes back long before the days of our Paleolithic ancestors. It reflects a deeper genetic heritage that pre-dates the very origin of primates, and was apparently retained throughout their evolution.

However, the hypothetical use of animal food by our primate ancestors must be placed into proper perspective. How much flesh food do modern anthropoids eat? Overall, very little. The apes that most closely resemble humans are the bonobos, chimpanzees, and gorillas. Chimpanzees have been seen extracting termites from holes in the tree, by using a saliva-moistened twig (which no doubt, pleases the tree). They have also been seen hunting and killing small mammals on occasion — a fact that is sometimes used by some dietary authors to suggest that humans are natural flesh eaters. However, this too needs to be placed in proper perspective. According to the observations of famed primatologist Jane Goodall, chimps often chew animal flesh along with leaves to extract the juice, and then, usually discard the residue. This would suggest that their capacity to digest animal products is limited. Regarding our own dietary needs, this behavior might also serve to remind us that the strong alkalizing power of vegetables is important to balance out the strongly acidifying influence of animal flesh.

Gorillas are too heavy to efficiently navigate through trees, so they eat mostly leaves and shoots — a fact that has been frequently used by vegetarian writers to support the idea that humans can be strong and healthy without consuming animal products. However, here again, the supposed vegan life-style of the gorilla must be put into proper perspective. Unlike most human vegans of today, gorillas rely on massive amounts of raw vegetation for the bulk of their calories — not cooked grains and beans! Regarding flesh food, gorillas have not been seen intentionally eating it, but neither have they been seen fastidiously cleaning insects and aphids from their veggies, as modern humans tend to do. It is conceivable that the tiny amount of incidental insects provides gorillas with needed nutrients. All this should be taken into consideration by those who wish to use the gorilla as a role model of a successful vegan.

Bonobos are our closest living anthropoid relatives. They are significantly more human-like than chimps, based on their anatomy, genetics, and behavior. How much flesh food do they eat? Very little, based on stool analysis. Their consumption of animal products seems to be somewhere between chimps and gorillas.[1]

Primate Paradise

One fascinating feature of the anthropoid life-style is their enjoyment of leisure time. Granted, the process of finding trees loaded with ripe fruit does require quite a bit of physical exercise. However, once they locate the banana bonanza or fig feast, their food is nutritious enough to eliminate the need to spend all their waking hours eating or searching for more food.

Modern anthropoids often spend hours "grooming" each other, wherein they sit around, picking and eating insects and debris from each other's skin. In other words, fruit provides the main course, and the bugs plucked from each other provide the dessert. We may also assume that part of their "dessert" is the emotional comfort and sense of security of gently touching one another. As with other big-brained mammals, anthropoids require physical touch, affection, and close social bonds. The bigger the brain, the greater the need for physical touch and emotional closeness.

Seems like a blissful life. Think of it. You eat fruit until full, and then lounge around, shaded from the hot sun, and protected from predators below, as you lovingly massage each other in the quiet of the afternoon, serenaded by song birds, as the tropical breeze cools you down. For the anthropoid ape, the tree is no less than an all-providing, omnipotent God. For the tree, the anthropoids are as ministering angels.

Paradise Lost

We might imagine that our anthropoid ancestors would have been perfectly happy to stay perched on their branches, munching on fruit, and grooming each other. However, that was not to be. We don't exactly when, but somewhere in time, our ancestors descended from the trees.[2] Why? The current accepted theory is that around 5 million years ago, the climate in Africa started changing. It became drier, consequently the vast tropical forests gradually thinned out.

Another intriguing possibility is that some of the anthropoid apes continued evolving into bigger and more efficient fruit eaters, even while trees were still abundant, and therefore, might have found it more convenient to spend more time on the ground.[3,4] This seems to be pretty much what happened to the gorilla.

Furthermore, as the brains of our ancestors continued to grow, babies had to be born sooner, so as to be able to fit through the birth canal. Consequently, infants were more helpless and required more care. Under such circumstances, the ability to stand and walk efficiently, with your arms free, is most advantageous.[5]

Regardless of what actually drove them down from trees, natural selection would have favored anthropoids that could stand straighter and walk faster. This allowed them to evade predators, as well as conserve energy — walking erect with an even stride is energetically more efficient than stooping forward and waddling like a duck. Through time, the legs became longer and the pelvis changed to allow for a more erect posture. Eventually, they crossed the threshold, transforming into a whole new breed of primates, which scientists call Hominids.

The Family of Man

Within the order of primates are a number of smaller groups or *families*. One such family is that of the Hominids, so called because of their close resemblance to modern humans. We are the only surviving hominids. However, if we were to encounter one of the early hominids, we might experience a sort of culture shock, and might be forced to reconsider what it means to be human.

The large and complex brain of the early hominids gave them the ability to learn from watching other animals. We might imagine them looking at a wart hog digging up starchy roots and tubers, thus giving the Hominids the idea of doing the same thing with a sharp stick. They may have been inspired by a predator or scavenger using its powerful jaw and teeth to crack open bones to get to the nutritious marrow. The hominoids' jaws and teeth were not suited for that, but our ancestors were apparently smart enough to do the same thing with a stone. Using the same technology, they could have also split open rotted logs to expose swarms of termites and grubs. Standing at the water's edge, holding a sharp stick, they may have watched an aquatic bird plucking a fish out of the water, and thought to themselves, "Hey, we can do that too!"

These are all plausible theories, but according to the dental analysis of early Hominids, they all seemed to prefer fruit, regardless of their emerging specializations and technologies — even though fruit trees were supposedly on the decline.[6] This may seem puzzling, until we remember that they probably learned how to take full advantage of the fruits that *were* available, perhaps using their emerging stick-and-stone technology to pick the trees clean. In other words, compared to the other fruit-eating animals, they had top priority over the food supply, by virtue of their size and smarts.

However, over time, the continued decline in the fruit supply would have necessitated that they use more of the other foods. Evolution continued to transform them in the direction of greater efficiency for walking and running. Their body-hair thinned out, so they could dissipate heat through sweating, thus allowing them to walk and run for extended periods under the hot sun. Meanwhile, the brain became even bigger, allowing them to further refine their skills for living on the ground.

And so, it came to pass that the tool user became a serious toolmaker. They had evolved into a new creature that was not merely in the same family as modern humans, but part of the smaller inner circle called Homo, which literally means "Man."

Food and Exponential Brain Growth

My fascination with human evolution began in high school, where I often neglected my required schoolwork, because I was devouring every evolution book I could get my hands on. I quickly became familiar with what was then one of the greatest mysteries in the science of paleontology, as illustrated in figure 7.1.

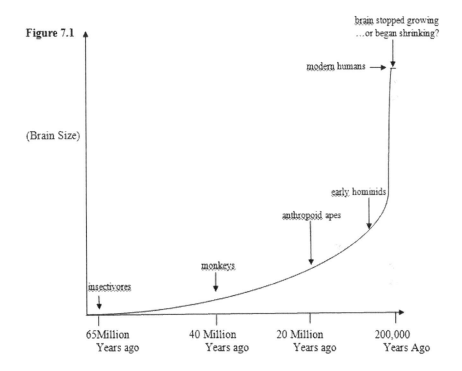

What is the big mystery? The preceding graph shows that around three million years ago, something extraordinary happened. The brains of our ancestors seemed to have more than doubled in size in a ridiculously short period of time (shown by the nearly vertical line, indicting brain growth), thus transforming early hominids into modern humans. Then, about 200,000 years ago, brain growth came to a screeching halt. In fact, according to some theories, the brain actually started shrinking!

What is it that compelled this extremely rapid growth? And why did it suddenly stop? To this day, that mystery is still a mystery.

Part of the brain mystery is the role played by food. Not surprisingly, dietary authors who favor a diet with a significant amount of animal products favor the idea that meat contributed to brain growth, while those who favor a plant-based diet say otherwise.

However, the inclusion of such evolutionary data to justify any diet can add even more confusion to an already confusing topic. Why? Nutritional authors are not paleontologists. Likewise, paleontologists are not nutrition specialists.[7] The result can be more confusing than the blind leading the blind. This is another reason to seriously question what *all* authorities have to say about the diet of our early ancestors — and its implication for our current nutritional needs.

For example, for most of the 20th century, paleontologists suggested that higher levels of animal fat and protein may have contributed to brain development. This is a reasonable hypothesis because the extremely rapid brain-growth at the dawn of humanity seems to coincide with an increase in the consumption of animal flesh.

The meat-theory of brain-growth has been used by the proponents of the modern Paleolithic Diet, which recommends that we get 50% of our calories from meat, and 50% from plant foods, as described in chapter 9. However, recent evidence suggests that the amount of flesh-food consumed by our Paleolithic ancestors may have been much lower.[8]

Furthermore, until recently, paleontologists did not consider the critically important role of plant nutrients, such as the antioxidants, for supporting the brain. Looking at the basic nutritional needs of the brain, carbohydrates provide the fuel that powers the brain cells, while protein and fat are the primary building materials. Less obvious but equally important, are the vitamins, minerals, and phytonutrients, which provide the regulatory functions, such as antioxidant activity, without which brain cells are rapidly destroyed by oxidation.

It is understandable that early paleontologists did not take into account the importance of plant chemicals for the brain, because the nutritional researchers of the day had not yet addressed such information. It is also understandable that paleontologists once assumed that our Paleolithic ancestors ate a lot of meat, because that is the sort of evidence that tends to leave the best artifacts (bones and stones). In contrast, the artifacts that point to the consumption of plant foods are more difficult to locate, especially as we go further back in time. It has only been in recent years that the science of paleontology has had the tools to see such evidence.

How much meat did our Paleolithic ancestors eat? And what role did it play in exponential brain growth? The mystery is more mysterious than ever — and has within it a puzzling contradiction.

The Contradiction

The contradiction becomes clear when we look at figure 7.1. The graph shows that the overall story of primate evolution is one of a small-brained insect eater transforming into a large-brained fruit eater. In other words, for tens of millions of years, brain growth in the evolving primates coincided with a *decrease* in the consumption of animal fat and protein, and an increase in fruit!

Is the association of large brain and a fruit diet a mere coincidence, unique to the primate lineage? Apparently not. Large brain size is a feature seen in other animals that utilize fruit as the primary source of calories. For example, fruit bats have a bigger brain than insect-eating bats. Fruit-eating parrots have such a big brain and display such keen intelligence that zoologists have jokingly bestowed upon them the title of "honorary primates."

Regarding primates, the relationship between fruit and the evolving brain is dramatized in a study done on two groups of monkeys: The spider monkey feasts on fruit, and the howler monkey eats mostly leaves. The leaf-eating monkeys tend to be slow, reserved, and passive. The fruit-eating monkeys have a larger brain and behave like typical primates — lively, curious, playful, and often mischievous.[9]

How are we to navigate through this complex maze of information? The answer: very carefully! With regard to the big brain in fruit-eating animals, it is still not clear if brain development is somehow assisted by the nutrients in the fruit, or simply represents a necessity for the procurement of fruit. Furthermore, as suggested in figure 7.1, the explosively fast brain growth at the dawn of humanity far exceeds the steady brain growth of the preceding 60 million years of primate evolution.

To further cloud the issue, it is tempting to want to fill in the gaps in our knowledge with our own pet theories and beliefs — especially for those who favor a particular dietary system. However, if our goal is to discover the truth, we should be cautious about making *any* assumptions, one way or the other. The fruit-brain connection does not preclude the possibility that increased meat consumption somehow contributed to the explosively fast brain-growth of early humans, but rather should compel us to regard the meat-theory with caution.

Fire and Food

The use of fire by our early ancestors is another arguing point among some of the dietary authors — especially in recent years, with the rise in popularity of the raw diets. From a strictly evolutionary standpoint, most paleontologists agree that our ancestors' access to fire and cooked food had a profound effect on their cultural and perhaps biological evolution.

Imagine what it might have been like. The one-time object of terror became a source of seemingly unlimited power. One of the effects of cooking is that it significantly increases the caloric value of food — especially plant food. And, that was just the beginning. Fire dispelled the chill and dangers of the night. The cave was no longer a place where they could be trapped by wandering predators. Instead, they were able to banish the bear from its cave, and thereby take up residence, so that we, their descendants, would one day come to know them as "Cave Men."

For the first time, they were able to relax after a long day, without having to fear predators lurking in the night. What an eerie feeling that must have been for those early humans, who otherwise had to be constantly vigilant. It may have given them a feeling of serenity that was new, but somehow familiar, perhaps evoking an ancient memory; an echo of their anthropoid ancestors, sitting safely in their arboreal perch, their bellies full, as they quietly groomed each other after a fruit meal, in the safety and security of the canopy.

With regard to nutrition, fire has other benefits besides increasing calories. It liberates other nutrients locked up in plant fiber. It warms and softens animal flesh, root vegetables, and grains. However, we now know that fire also destroys nutrients, including some vitamins and many phytonutrients, while altering proteins, fats, and carbohydrates in ways that create toxic chemicals, including some potent carcinogens. Therefore, if our goal is optimum health and longevity, an important question emerges. How well adapted are we to eating cooked food?

According to current estimates, the time period for the earliest use of fire ranges from two million to 125,000 years ago, though most scientists seem to favor a date of about 230,000 years.[10] Either way, given the relatively recent use of fire, the question regarding our biological adaptation to cooked food is a legitimate one. The dramatic increase in meat consumption after tens of millions of years of the primate diet is radical enough, but the sudden inclusion of cooked food is even more radical. In fact, it is unprecedented in the history of life on Earth!

How has the cooking (and mixing) of food affected a biological system that has been adapted for hundreds of millions of years to accept food that is fresh, raw, and typically eaten one at a time? Granted, some biological adaptation to cooked food may have occurred. However, that still doesn't necessarily mean cooked food is nutritionally superior or even equivalent to raw food — especially for the big brain, which is extremely rich in omega-3 fats and has a very high metabolic rate, both of which create a great need for the phytonutrients and antioxidants present in raw fruits and vegetables. It may certainly be argued that the drastic reduction in these brain-protecting raw plant nutrients and replacing them with high-calorie cooked food (with large amounts of oxidized fats and other toxins), could have adversely affected the body and mind.

Not surprisingly, those dietary systems that use a significant amount of cooked food (which is most of them) tend to downplay the possible toxic and nutrient-destroying effects of cooking, while perhaps asserting or implying that fire has been part of the human experience long enough to allow for some adaptation. Likewise, proponents of diets that are high in raw foods emphasize the detrimental effects of cooking.

The Mysterious Paleolithic Period

Whatever the factors that provided the final push for the emergence of the modern human brain, our ancestors did apparently become fully human during the estimated two million years of the Paleolithic Period. They completely populated Africa, and, at least on two separate occasions, migrated northward.

First Wave

The first exodus out of Africa happened before the emergence of modern humans. They populated the Mid-East, and then on to Asia and Europe. The early humans who first populated Asia are called Homo erectus. The first Europeans are the ones we call the Neanderthals. The ones that stayed in Africa eventually became us.

The Neanderthals in Europe had to endure the ice age, so they became hunters of mammoth and other big game. In Africa, the weather was warmer, but life was not much easier, because the climate had become very dry. Apparently, our African ancestors hunted, fished, and gathered fruit and vegetables, including starchy vegetables and grains.

Dietary systems that favor the liberal use of animal products have pointed to the Neanderthals to support the safety of a high-meat diet. However, more recent evidence suggests that Neanderthals consumed a significant amount of plant food, including cooked starchy foods.[11]

Even if Neanderthals did eat mostly meat, we should be cautious about applying such data to our own needs, because survival is not the same as optimum health. For example, the high levels of heme-iron in meat can generate a significant amount of oxidative stress, which has been linked to Alzheimer's disease and other forms of neurodegeneration.[12] This, apparently, did not stop the Neanderthals from reproducing and raising their children, but could have hindered cognitive function and shortened their lives.

On that note, some paleontologists believe that fish in the diet of our ancestors in Africa gave them a brain-boosting edge over the Neanderthals in Europe. However, to properly apply this information to our own modern needs, we must, again, keep in mind that the brain does not live by fat and protein alone. The high metabolic rate and large amount of fat in the brain (especially the extremely sensitive DHA), requires strong antioxidant protection, without which the brain cells rapidly die from oxidative stress, especially on a diet that includes significant amounts of cooked meat.

Furthermore, the same plant foods that provide antioxidants also provide the alkalizing power that balances the acidifying influence of cooked animal flesh and grains. Greater alkalizing power and antioxidant protection can translate into a potentially longer life span, with a brain that remains sharper into later years, allowing each individual to gather more knowledge and share it with the next generation. This might, at least partially, explain why our ancestors' tools, clothing, and artwork were more elaborate compared to that of Neanderthals.

In addition, we also now know that the alkalizing power of fruits and vegetables is important to keep bones strong. Modern human societies (traditional and industrialized) that consume a great deal of animal flesh, with little fruits and vegetables, consistently show a higher incidence of osteoporosis and hip fractures. The message for modern humans is clear: If you eat significant amounts of meat, make sure you also get an ample amount of vegetables and fruit.

Second Wave

The second exodus out of Africa is estimated to have occurred about 70,000 years ago. Some of our African ancestors (fully modern, by then) migrated northward again. Their migration into Asia marked the end of Homo erectus. Their migration into Europe marked the end of the Neanderthals.

Then, about 12,000 years ago, the climate finally became wetter and warmer. The skills that our ancestors had honed in order to survive the lean times, would allow them to not just survive, but also flourish. However, their great success meant their time as hunter-gatherers was coming to an end.

The Neolithic Revolution

The first evidence of cultivation is that of fig trees in the Mid-East, about 13,000 years ago. That is not surprising. Up to that point, our ancestors had been consuming fruit longer and more consistently than any other food — with figs being a favorite among primates. However, it was the widespread cultivation of grains, about 10,000 years ago, that radically changed the lives of our ancestors.

An abundance of grains gave our ancestors a stable food supply all year round. Cultivated grains also facilitated the domestication of animals and the introduction of dairy.

The relative abundance of calorically rich food resulted in an unprecedented growth in the human population. However, here we can pose another nutritional question. Was the shift from eating fruits/vegetables/meat to grains/beans/dairy a change for the better or worse? This is yet another area of disagreement among the various dietary systems described in chapter 9.

On the one hand, there are reasons to believe that grains are not perfect food:
- Since grains seem to have been cultivated just 10,000 years ago, it has been argued that humans are not well adapted to consume them in large quantities.
- The skeletons of the Neolithic farmers suggest they were not as big, robust, and healthy as their hunter/gatherer ancestors.
- Today, the over-consumption of grains is associated with some degenerative diseases, such as arthritis.
- Compared with fruits and vegetables, grains are higher in calories but lower in vitamins, minerals, and phytonutrients. Grains also contain some chemicals, such as phytate, which could pull some minerals out of the body.

On the other hand, grains don't look so bad when we look at the bigger picture:
- Even though grains and starchy vegetables are different from fruit, they still have a nutritional profile that is more akin to fruit, compared to animal products.

- Many cultures have, through the centuries, found ways of making grains and dairy less problematical and more digestible and nutritious, through soaking, sprouting, kneading, and fermentation.
- Though 10,000 years ago is cited as the time that our ancestors started to seriously settle down and rely on cultivated plants, there is evidence that starchy vegetables and grains may have been a significant part of the human diet as far back as 105,000 years.[13] Furthermore, such evidence does not fossilize as readily as bones and stone tools, therefore, it is hard to say just how long ago humans started to seriously rely on starchy foods.

Adaptation to Non-primate Foods

Here are a few other signs that some biological adaptation did occur:
- DNA studies have shown that humans have more genes that code for the starch-digesting enzyme compared to chimps. This suggests that starchy foods have been a significant food in the human lineage far longer than suggested by the previously collected fossil evidence.
- Compared to apes, humans retain more uric acid in the body. Meat tends to increase the level of uric acid in the body, suggesting an adaptation to this food.
- Humans can refrain from eating for several days without experiencing harmful consequences. In fact, under the right conditions, we can fast for a month or longer. Apes can't do that. We can fast because we store more fat. When we fast, we burn a lot of that fat, which results in the production of organic molecules called ketones. Technically, ketones are the result of the inefficient and incomplete combustion of fats. Though ketones are toxic in large amounts, humans can apparently tolerate them better than apes. Furthermore, our brain cells can actually burn ketones for energy, in place of glucose, if dietary carbohydrates are severely restricted.

On the Other Hand...

Our capacity to fast and utilize ketones has been used by proponents of low-carb diets to support the idea that humans evolved on a high-meat and high-fat diet. This is valid hypothesis, but does not *prove* that our ancestors ate a lot of fat. The capacity to fast could very well be an adaptation to periods of less food or no food – of *any* kind.

With regard to the current dietary debates, the bottom line is this: Those who advocate a high-meat diet assert that humans have been eating animal foods far too long to just give it up without negative consequences. On the other hand, proponents of vegetarian and vegan diets point to the studies that show an increase in degenerative diseases with increased consumption of animal products, and therefore promote starchy foods as the main source of calories.

However, closer examination suggests that neither grains nor meat qualify as ideal foods for modern humans — in very large amounts, at least. Two clues that support this idea have to do with vitamin A and vitamin C.

Vitamin A and Vitamin C

True carnivores do not make vitamin A (retinol), reflecting an abundance of this vitamin in their diet. In contrast, plant-eating animals (including primates) make vitamin A from the beta-carotene, found abundantly in fruits and vegetables. The persistence of the ability to make vitamin A in modern humans (including Eskimos) is yet another indicator that we come from a long line of fruit-and-vegetables eaters, and that any hypothetical adaptation to animal products (or grains, for that matter) is limited.[13]

Granted, the conversion rate of beta-carotene to vitamin A is low (4-27%.)[14] This fact has been used by some nutritional authors to suggest that humans are dependent on animal products — which are the only reliable sources of pre-formed vitamin A. However, with the typical primate diet, rich in fresh fruits and vegetables, the conversion of beta-carotene to vitamin A does not have to be efficient, especially when we consider that one molecule of beta-carotene converts into two molecules of vitamin A. The low conversion rate is a problem only if we are consuming the typical modern diet that is dominated by cooked grains and deficient in fruits and vegetables. With such a diet, animal products or supplements are needed to supply adequate amounts of vitamin A.

The situation with vitamin C is even more revealing. The vast majority of animals make their own vitamin C. Primates, including humans, are among the few exceptions. Apparently, tropical fruit and wild greens provide such a rich supply of vitamin C that all primates have long ago lost the ability to produce it. This point is particularly significant when we consider that vitamin C requirements in all animals are quite high, as described in chapter 3. Even grazing animals, which get a substantial amount of vitamin C from food, still have to make it internally.

What is the point? The point is that humans apparently did not "resurrect" the ability to make vitamin C during the Paleolithic Period, even though the consumption of fruits and vegetables was supposedly greatly reduced in favor of cooked animal products and starchy foods — poor sources of vitamin C. This raises a question to which I alluded earlier: How much meat did our Paleolithic ancestors actually eat — and for how long? The fact that we retained a dietary dependency on vitamin C suggests that the consumption of raw fruits and vegetables might have remained quite high for a major part of the Paleolithic Period. Either that or their health seriously declined.

Granted, our higher levels uric acid, and our capacity to fast and utilize ketones suggests that some adaptation did occur to a non-primate diet. Also, our ancestors obviously did survive well enough to populate the Earth. However, survival is not the same as optimum health. Our continued dependence on dietary vitamin C suggests that our physiological adaptation to a diet dominated by cooked meat, grains, and starchy tubers was modest, at best.

Alternate Theories of Human Evolution

Before we conclude this romp through the history and prehistory of human nutrition, I would like to point out that the information regarding our prehistoric ancestors is not set in stone – so to speak. The last "t" has not been crossed, and the last "i" has not been dotted regarding who we are, and where we came from.

The more closely we examine the Paleolithic Period, the more mysterious it seems. The data include gaps, tantalizing puzzles, and anomalies that have invited alternate theories of human origins. I mention them here because, if any of them turn out to have a measure of validity, they could radically alter the currently accepted model of human evolution —including the role played by food.

As an example, in contrast to the accepted model of human evolution, which assumes a steady upward progression, some of these alternative theories, in agreement with the creation myths and scriptures of various cultures, suggest that humans had a so-called "Golden Age" many thousands of years ago, during which they reached a zenith of biological and cultural development — and have been degenerating ever since![15] That Golden Age does not refer to the high culture of ancient Greece or China, 2-4 thousand years ago. By then, according to the writings of Plato, humanity was already deep into its decline. The Golden Age supposedly goes further back well into the Paleolithic Period.

Such stories stand in stark contrast to the popular image of Paleolithic humans as primitive brutes, gnawing on bones. These stories tell us that our distant ancestors were, for a long stretch of time, mostly or totally vegetarians, who lived longer and were healthier, smarter, and more peaceful than modern humans. They supposedly reached a level of sophistication, stability, and civility that is now, literally, mythical to us.[16]

The Fruit Theory

One alternate theory is especially relevant to nutrition because it proposes that our ancestors ate mostly fruit for most of Paleolithic Period! They supposedly did not become true hunter/gatherers until about 200,000 years ago.[17] Using this model, the explosively fast brain-growth at the dawn of the Paleolithic Period (figure 7.1) was simply an acceleration of the already rapid brain growth seen in arboreal primates — and was fueled by the same fruit-based diet![18]

According to the fruit theory, the wealth of phytonutrients (especially the flavonoids) found in fruit and other tropical plants, provided powerful regulatory roles that allowed the primate brain to grow faster and faster for tens of millions of years, culminating with the exponential brain growth that transformed early hominids into modern humans. If this theory has a measure of validity, our ancestors' alleged degeneration (metaphorically described as a "fall from grace") was triggered by a loss of their ancestral food.

The "fall" supposedly began when our ancestors had to rely more heavily on non-primate foods, starting around 200,000 years ago, and was aggravated by the increased reliance on cooked food. However, the physical and psychological degeneration took a major turn for the worse when they shifted from the hunter/gatherer lifestyle to grain farming. The latter idea is supported by archeological evidence that suggests humans became smaller and less healthy after they began relying heavily on cultivated grains.[19]

Epigenetics – Evolution in the Fast Lane

One reason that human origins have been puzzling is that, until recently, paleontologists did not know about epigenetics, a new field of study that is compelling scientists to rethink genetics and inheritance. Essentially, epigenetics says that the environment (especially food) can have a profound effect on gene expression. For example, the diet of the mother can powerfully influence genetic expression in the fetus.

Even more astounding (and downright shocking to biologists, when first discovered), is that the effects of food on gene expression do not merely impact the individual eating the food and their immediate offspring, but can be passed on to the future generations![20] What does this mean for evolution? It means that evolution can happen a lot faster than biologists previously thought.

Until recently, the idea that food eaten by parents can affect the genetic expression of the offspring has been largely ignored or actively dismissed by biologists and nutritional authors, because it was contrary to the so-called "central dogma" of biology, which basically says that genes determine everything — and that they are not subject to change, except through the slow process of random mutation.

The Weston A. Price Diet was the first dietary system that seriously considered the idea that the diet of the parents affects the offspring.[21] The fruit theory of human evolution goes one step further by suggesting that a diet of tropical fruits and vegetables drove the explosively fast evolution of the human brain (through epigenetic influences), and then, the subsequent loss of those foods started our gradual decline.

Mainstream paleontology and archeology still do not officially recognize any of the alternate theories. I do not necessarily accept them either, but neither have I seen evidence that would compel me to categorically reject any of them. The official story has too many unanswered questions and anomalies to casually dismiss the alternate theories. What seems far-fetched today may prove to be valid tomorrow. If the history of science has taught us anything, it has taught us that truth can turn out to be stranger than any fiction that we can spin.

Whether or not the fruit theory of human evolution has any validity, its assertions do include important nutritional information that is relevant to modern humans. Firstly, it reminds us that the phytonutrients of fruits and vegetables are vitally important for keeping the brain alive and well in the individual. Secondly, it points to the exciting epigenetic influences that such foods can have on the brain of the baby, reminding us that the diet of the mother does, indeed, have a profound effect on the development of the nervous system and general health of the in-utero baby.

The Big Picture

Whether we favor the mainstream or alternate theories of human origins, the big picture regarding the diets of our ancestors looks sort of like this:

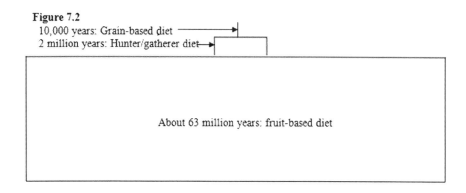

Figure 7.2
10,000 years: Grain-based diet
2 million years: Hunter/gatherer diet
About 63 million years: fruit-based diet

As suggested by figure 7.2, fruits and vegetables have been the dominant foods in the primate lineage far longer than any of the other food groups. However, *somewhere* within the last two million years, fruit consumption was apparently reduced in favor of cooked animal products, starchy vegetables, and grains. Then, about 10,000 years ago, humans began relying heavily on cultivated grains.

The Quest for Simplicity

Though we would like to have quick and simple answers, the big picture regarding our ancestors' diets, and the implications for modern humans, has some unanswered questions:

- Since we are the only animals that eat cooked food, and started doing so relatively recently, how adapted are we for this?
- Since our anatomy and physiology is fundamentally designed for the primate diet, how adapted are we to the large amounts of meat, dairy, grains, and starchy vegetables that dominate most modern diets?
- Have our ancestors been exiled from the "Garden" long enough to result in a significant altering of our fundamental fruitarian foundation? Has our capacity to metabolize fruit become "rusty?" Are some humans rustier than others? Are some humans not rusty at all?
- Do we need to consume protein, fat, and animal products in amounts exceeding the typical primate proportions?
- How do the fruits of today compare nutritionally to those of our ancestors?
- Beyond the evolutionary questions, how much can we generalize about the nutritional needs of modern humans? Is it "one size fits all," as many authors imply, or is there so much variation as to make generalization difficult, at best?

Conclusion — Eating Is Very Personal

Thankfully, some simple guidelines are emerging that can be of benefit to all individuals looking for their ideal diet. Nutritional studies throughout the world strongly suggest a need to honor our primate roots to a certain degree, even if our need for starchy foods and animal products does exceed primate proportions.[22] This is the take-home lesson for the student of nutrition.

Beyond that, regard *all* theories of human origins and diet with caution — avoid trying to justify your chosen diet by tightly clutching to certain theories of human origins. The current pool of information may be fascinating and even useful, but we must remember that it is subject to change.

With our collective genetic heritage, every one of us can claim, "I am a fruit eater, I am a meat eater, and I am a grain eater." These three patterns dance together in the body and mind of every human, because enough time has passed to allow all three to have become encoded in our genetic and epigenetic "primal blueprint," to a certain degree.

Furthermore, the dance seems to occur differently in every individual. This is why, in our quest for the ideal diet, we should be cautious about over-generalizing. What should *we* eat? This question seems to have no simple answer that applies to everyone. In my opinion, a more practical approach is to ask, What should *I* eat?

Chapter 8
How to Evaluate Any Diet

Limitations in the availability of some foods, diversity of preferences, and constitutional variations among humans have created fertile ground for the emergence of many dietary systems — and much disagreement among them. The proponents of Diet "A" warn us of the dangers of Diet "B" and vice versa. What's more, both parties might sound pretty convincing! When we also consider the deep emotions we tend to have with food, we can see how the disagreement can become rather heated.

The more emotional charge we have on food, the less objective we tend to be. This certainly applies to the individuals who teach a particular diet. No matter how intelligent and sincere the teachers, they will probably be less than totally objective. To complicate matters, there might also be a substantial financial investment. When money pressures demand that we "sell" our product, objectivity can easily fall by the wayside.

Those who promote a particular diet might emphasize the strong points and minimize the weak ones. Like the rest of us emotional humans, the diet teachers are often tempted to jump to conclusions and present opinion as fact, while censoring information that does not support their teachings. I certainly find myself tempted in this manner — even though I personally do not have financial ties to any one given system. I can only imagine how much more difficult it is for someone who does have such financial ties.

Food Fight

Controversy is a cheap and easy way to stand out. Battles tend to draw attention. The easiest way to look good is to make the other guy look bad. Granted, I can appreciate the need to honestly express perceived flaws or weak areas in any given diet, but when such expressions of "passion" takes the form of *argumentum ad hominem* (character attack), the accuser does a disservice to the seeker of health. I can also understand the need to use the emotional appeal to sell a product. Such strategies tend to produce quick results, but we do pay the price. We sacrifice truth for the sake of profit.

Such attacks on the competition are a source of confusion for the general public, not just because the presenters are fighting, but also because they frequently misrepresent each other. The diet teachers might be very knowledgeable about their respective diets, but their knowledge of the competition is often limited and their assessment is flawed.

Also, like the rest of us, they have a tendency to compare the strong points of their diet to the weak points in someone else's diet. They highlight what it best in their diet and what is worst in the competition — while ignoring the other side of the coin. They might do this unintentionally, but it is still a formula for endless war, and a source of confusion for the health-seeking public.

Hopefully, as consumers educate themselves and are better able to see past all this, the various vendors will learn that it is more advantageous to create a product that will endure and present it clearly and honestly. They will learn that, if indeed, their diet really does have value, the use of language that is conservative and rational wins out every time over sensationalism or aggression. They will learn that if their product really is any good, they can just focus their energy on presenting it honestly and effectively, rather diverting attention from its weaknesses by attacking the completion.

Expressing yourself aggressively will, at best, create a momentary dazzle that quickly burns out. Expressing with an attitude of inflated authority is likely to immediately turn off any serious researcher or health professional, while arousing suspicion (perhaps subconsciously) in the general reader.

I find that I am more receptive to authors who manage to be clear and direct, while minimizing criticism of other authors. I tend to trust authors who seem to have a sense of how their teachings relate with other ideas, rather than being quick to defend their territory. I cannot help but smile on the inside when I read information conveyed with language that seems to carry a higher vision — one that recognizes the natural harmony and complementarity between seemingly competing ideas.

The good news is that we do have solid nutritional information and useful dietary guidelines that anyone can benefit from. However, by the time the pure science reaches the public, it has already been filtered through teachers and writers who have a strong bias or vested interest in one dietary philosophy.

How do we navigate through this? The simple rule of thumb is to just get both sides of the story on any given dietary issue. The chapter that follows offers a survey of every major dietary system that is currently being promoted to the public. If any of these diets seriously speak to you, I suggest you do two things:

- Learn as much as you can from the teachers and advocates of the diet in question.
- Listen to what the critics have to say.

Yes, it is that simple. However, "simple" is not the same as "easy." In this case, the simple solution also requires that you endeavor to maintain the same measure of intellectual honesty and objectivity that you would expect from the diet teacher.

Do Not Marry Your Diet

Since objectivity is not necessarily as easy as we might think, let us give it some attention here. Objectivity can become increasingly difficult as we delve more deeply into one particular way of eating. With every book we read and seminar we attend, we insidiously become more indoctrinated and emotionally "imprinted." Eventually, we are no longer seekers of knowledge, but defenders of the faith.

This sort of behavior might seem strange to someone who is new to the study of nutrition. The beginner might declare, "That's silly, I would never do that!" However, since this sort of behavior seems to be more the rule than the exception among advocates of the various diets, the newbie should be mindful of it.

A given diet probably works well for the individuals who endorse it, therefore, they will, perhaps in all sincerity, say only good things about it. In fact, their passion and enthusiasm might be so contagious, that the listener becomes "converted." The result: objectivity falls by the wayside for everyone.

In other words, a given diet might work really well for a given individual, and this is the same person who gets excited about it, and spreads the word. We generally do not hear much from the people who have only fair or mediocre results.

The fundamental question is, how will the diet work for *you?* That is a question that only personal experience can answer. You can best answer it for yourself by being as objective as possible. Regardless of which dietary road you take, when you discipline yourself to remain fairly objective, you are likely to discover that most dietary systems have something of value to offer. You might even start to see how competing dietary systems are actually related — you start to connect the dots. In addition, though the study of nutrition can be complicated, you will discover that the basics are actually quite simple, as described below.

How Professionals Analyze Diets

The key to understanding any diet is to determine its caloric signature. By this, I am not referring to the mere counting of calories. Specifically, we must consider the ratio of calories provided by carbohydrates, protein, and fat in a given food. This is how scientists and dietitians analyze diets. To illustrate this, take a look at the table below, showing the caloric analysis of various foods:

Name	% Carbs	% Protein	% Fats
Fruits	90	5	5
Vegetables	70	15	15
Whole wheat	80	5	15
Most legumes	75	5	20
Peanuts	11	73	16
Walnuts	8	84	8
Ground beef	0	65	35
Lamb	0	75	25
Chicken	0	55	45
Pork	0	51	49
Fish	1	52	47
Whole milk	30	49	21
Mozzarella cheese	3	66	31

A brief examination of the above table reveals a pattern. In general, naturally occurring foods that tend to be higher in fat are proportionately lower in carbohydrates. For example, animal products, nuts, and seeds provide calories mostly from fat, and little, if any, from carbohydrates. On the other hand, fruits, vegetables, whole grains, and beans tend to be high in carbohydrates and relatively low in fat. In other words, *whole foods, in their natural form, generally feature either carbohydrates or fats as the dominant source of calories.* The two have an inverse relationship. As one goes up, the other goes down — like a seesaw.[1]

What Should I Eat?

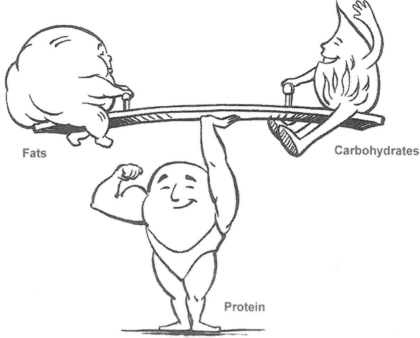

(From The 80-10-10 Diet by Dr. Douglas Graham)

How We Go Off Track

Once we recognize the seesaw relationship of carbohydrates and fats in whole foods, we can easily see the fundamental problem with many processed foods. Quite simply, we mix substantial amounts of high-carb foods and high-fat foods — pizza, hamburgers, cookies, cakes, candy, ice cream, etc. Consuming large amounts of these foods can precipitate a number of problems, such as indigestion, blood sugar issues, overeating, and obesity.

Not surprisingly, most of the major diets discussed in the next chapter attempt to resolve this issue by lowering either fats or carbohydrates. It seems to work — at least in the short term. Many common health issues improve, simply by avoiding the clash of these two caloric titans.

Looking at the Numbers

The National Institute of Health (NIH) recommends that 55-60% of daily calories come from carbohydrates, no more than 30% from fats, and

10-15% from protein. The World Health Organization (WHO) offers similar numbers. Though many dietary teachers deviate from these proportions, the NIH and WHO guidelines still provide a useful reference point for evaluating and comparing various diets, as shown in the table below.

Name	% of Carbs	% of Protein	% of Fat
NIH	55–60	10–15	< 30
Low-fat Diets	60–80	10–15	10–20
Low-carb Diets	10–40	15–30	40–70

In the above table, you will notice that diets deviate from NIH by either reducing the fat or carbohydrates. In other words, whether you are aware of it or not, your ideal diet will, first and foremost, get you into your ideal "zone," where your body is getting the proper ratio of carbohydrates, fats, and protein.

That ratio, in my opinion, can vary from person to person, and may not necessarily have to be very precise for a given individual. It can even vary with the seasons. Nonetheless, most nutritional authors would agree there is an ideal zone in which your body prefers to get its calories.

Granted, there is disagreement as to where to place the borders of that zone, but, when you chronically go too far beyond *your* ideal zone, the body will experience predictable problems — sooner or later.

My point here is not to favor low-carb or low-fat diets, but rather to emphasize that the proportion of carbohydrates, fats, and protein is the scientific foundation for understanding *any* diet. When this foundation has been established, we can make sense of the other considerations. Without this foundational knowledge, confusion reigns, or we have to blindly trust the creators of a given diet.

Do I Really Have to Know This Calorie Stuff?

The simple answer is no — provided you have enough access to your eating instincts. However, when your food radar is not working as well as you would like, the understanding of calories gives you a map that helps you find your way back to your ideal diet.

In other words, the main reason we even need such a map is that our food instincts (especially the sense of taste) are exposed to foods and combinations of foods not found in nature. The more we alter and mix foods, the tougher it is for our sense of taste to distinguish nutrients from toxins, or to determine when the body had eaten enough. For example, the common practice of mixing large quantities high-carb foods with high-fat foods, as with a cheese burger, French fries, and soft drink, will just about guarantee that we will have over-consumed calories by the time we feel "full." This is where a map can be very useful.

With such a map, you can easily recognize a diet's caloric signature, regardless of how it is marketed. Beyond that, another way to keep things simple is to remember that you choose only for yourself. You do not have to conform with your neighbor or vice versa.

The main purpose of this chapter is to present the basics about the caloric map. The next chapter will guide you in becoming proficient in reading the map, so you can make sense of where you are going on your nutritional journey.

Chapter 9
Survey of Major Diets

- Low-carb Diets
- Low-fat Diets
- Crossover Diets
- Raw Diets

The majority of the diets described in this chapter are either low-carb or low-fat, including the raw diets. The rest of them, I call the crossover diets, because they attempt to be somewhat "neutral," or they provide both low-carb and low-fat options.

Low-carb Diets

The low-carbohydrate diets are typically high in fat. Most of them rely on animal products for the bulk of daily calories, although, more recently, low-carb diets are emerging that provide for more plant-based foods.

On the positive side, low-carb diets greatly reduce or eliminate refined grains, sugar, and trans-fats, as well as facilitating weight loss. What are the long-term effects of such a diet? Good question. The modern low-carb diets have not been around that long. Several studies do indicate that low-carb diets are associated with a higher overall mortality rate, compared to the general population, but these must be considered as preliminary.[1] These studies do not "prove" anything, but point the way for further investigation. For example, most of these studies do not distinguish between low-carb diets that emphasize plant foods, and those that emphasize animal foods, as the primary source of calories. One study does make the distinction, and found that individuals on a low-carb diet with a high percentage of plant foods showed a lower overall mortality rate compared with the general population.[2]

However, whether or not the above studies turn out to be meaningful, meat-based low-carb diets do have several features that are cause for concern:

- Fats and protein, in general, require more digestive effort and cleanup, compare with carbohydrates, but this is especially true for fats and protein from animal sources. For example, animal protein tends to be more strongly acidifying than plant protein, due to the higher sulfur content. This is particularly significant when we remember that animal products, especially red meat, have a much higher levels protein, compared to plant foods.
- Though the role of high levels of saturated fats and cholesterol in cardiovascular disease has been questioned in recent years, oxidized cholesterol has been shown to damage to the walls of arteries.[3] Since meat is generally cooked (often at high temperatures) large amounts of it could expose the body to a steady bombardment of oxidized cholesterol. Appendix D describes this issue in more detail.
- Animal flesh, especially red meat, tends to have high levels of heme iron, which we cannot regulate as well as plant derived iron. High levels of heme iron can accelerate the oxidation of cholesterol. Heme iron also oxidizes delicate brain chemicals, leading to Alzheimer's disease and other neurodegenerative diseases. Diets featuring high levels of animal protein have been associated with increased incidence of Alzheimer's disease.[4]
- Studies suggest that high levels of animal protein create an excess of branched chain amino acids in the blood, which contribute to insulin resistance.[5]
- The so-called "high quality" or "complete" protein found in animal products is cited as a positive feature of animal products. However, in large amounts, such protein significantly raises levels of IGF-1 (insulin-like growth factor-1), which is associated with increased risk of cancer, cardiovascular disease, type II diabetes, rapid aging, and reduced lifespan.[6]
- True carnivores generally eat one big meal, and then abstain from food for a few days. This is probably similar to how our Paleolithic ancestors ate meat. No animal in the wild eats meat three times a day, as is often done with modern low-carb diets.

In addition to the above issues, eating substantially more protein and fat than the body needs, can predispose the individual to other metabolic stresses. As you may recall, the breakdown of protein produces ammonia, a potent metabolic poison, which, among other things, seriously irritates the kidneys. The breakdown of large amounts of fats produces ketones, resulting in the acidification of the blood, and irritates the kidneys. These issues are reduced by adequate levels of carbohydrates in the diet, which tend to inhibit the breakdown of protein and fat, thus minimizing the production of ammonia and ketones.[7]

The question is, *how much* fat and protein is too much? For example, higher levels of dietary fat and protein have been linked with insulin resistance, but how high is too high? And, how low do the dietary carbohydrates have to be before we lose their protective protein-sparing and ketone lowering effects? Opinions vary. Furthermore, the question of individual differences is usually ignored or actively dismissed.

In general, those who advocate low-carb diets believe the average person can safely consume more protein and fat than recommended by the NIH and WHO, and that higher levels of ketones are safe. Meanwhile, those who promote low-fat diets generally set the tolerance levels much lower.

Regarding fat, we have another point to consider. The studies linking high-fat diets with degenerative diseases typically focus on *quantity*, not *quality*. Proponents of low-carb diets assert that quality does make a difference. How big of a difference? When additional data is available, we might be able to say something more definitive on this issue. However, for now, it is reasonable to suggest that a high-fat diet featuring the proper amounts of omega-3 and omega-6 oils, with a goodly amount of plant-based fats from whole food sources is going to be easier on the body than one overloaded with oxidized cholesterol, trans-fats, and extracted oils.

The Atkins Diet

The Atkins Diet was the first of the modern low-carb diets. The original version of this diet advises the individual to consume large amounts of animal products, while avoiding grains, starchy vegetables, and fruit.

Caloric Ratio: Carbs 5-30% Protein 25-30% Fats 55-70%

Strong Points
- It is doable for the average person. All foods are readily available.
- It provides the same benefits of most low-carb diets: rapid weight loss and even rapid improvement in blood pressure, blood lipids, and blood sugar.

Weak Points and Criticisms

- In the original version of the diet, little attention was given to quality of food. For example, the individual was advised to drink cream sweetened with aspartame.
- As shown by the caloric ratio, the level of carbohydrates can be extremely low, necessitating very high levels of protein and fat that can stress the kidneys and liver.
- There have been numerous reports of illness on this diet, including some lawsuits.
- It can have the long-term harmful effects associated with excessive levels of protein and fat described in the previous chapter. For example, the initial improvement in blood pressure and blood lipids is sometimes followed by a worsening of both.[8]
- Dr. Akins died of a heart attack, supposedly from complications from a fall. However, at the time of death, he was clinically obese, and his family refused to have an autopsy done.

Some of the issues associated with this diet are addressed by simply selecting higher quality food, reducing the animal products, and replacing them with generous servings of vegetables and fruit. In fact, the revised version of the Atkins Diet does just that, to a certain extent. The two low-carb diets described below go even further.

The Weston A. Price Diet

This diet is said to be based on research done by Dr. Weston A. Price in the 1930s. He traveled the world, and noticed people were significantly healthier when they lived on traditional diets consisting of locally grown or wild foods.

Though the cultures studied by Dr. Price varied widely in the foods they ate, the creators of this diet believe there is enough of a pattern to use Dr. Price's findings to promote their own dietary recommendations, which may be summarized as follows: A liberal amount of animal flesh, dairy, eggs, vegetables, fermented products, and a modest amount of whole grains, legumes, and fruit.

Caloric Ratio: Carbs 10-35% Protein 20-30% Fats 45-65%

Strong Points
- Offers a wide variety of foods, and is therefore very doable.
- Promotes locally grown foods and sustainable agriculture, such as organic and biodynamic farming.[9]
- The use of animal products includes raw milk, pasture-raised animals, free-range poultry, and their eggs.
- This diet discourages the consumption of foods that come from animals raised in unsanitary and inhumane factory farms.
- This diet discourages the overconsumption of refined sugar, grains, and highly processed soy products, and strongly discourages the consumption any GMO foods.
- This diet encourages individuals to reduce highly-processed packaged foods, and to learn the art of preparing clean and nutritious foods at home, such as traditional sourdough bread.
- The Weston A. Price Foundation provides instruction on how to use the whole animal, including organ meats and soup stocks made from bone and bone marrow, as our agricultural ancestors used to do.
- The Weston A. Price Foundation provides instruction on how to make high quality fermented products at home, especially cultured vegetables, to promote digestion, improve nutritional profile of foods, and reduce the presence of toxins and antinutrients in the foods. These foods also help to correct imbalances in intestinal bacteria, which can happen when large amounts of fat and protein are consumed.

Weak Points and Criticisms
- Some critics of this diet claim that the cultures studied by Dr. Price varied too widely in their diets to justify using his name to describe this particular dietary system.
- Dr. Price did not track the subjects of his study for an extended period of time.
- As a dentist, he focused mainly on teeth and dental arches, giving little attention to the rest of the body. Nor did he give much consideration to longevity. For example, he supposedly praised the meat-and-dairy-consuming Maasai of Africa for their robust physique and vitality, but apparently was not aware of their short lifespan and high incidence of osteoporosis.[10]

- Some critics claim that the actual diet that was ultimately recommended by Dr. Price was lower in fat and protein, and used animal products conservatively, contrary to the recommendations of the modern Weston A. Price Diet.[11]

The Paleolithic Diet

Like the previous diet, the Paleolithic Diet provides a substantial amount of calories from animal products. The main difference is the Paleo Diet uses less fat, and makes an effort to reduce the saturated fat.

Caloric Ratio: Carbs 22-40% Protein 20-35% Fats 28-47%

This diet establishes its essential features by using lean meats and an abundance of low-starch vegetables, and some fruits, especially the lower-glycemic fruits, such as berries. Eggs are permitted in moderation. The original version of the diet excludes dairy, grains, legumes, and potatoes.

A more recent variation on this diet is the **Primal Diet**, which provides 50-60% of calories from fat, does not restrict saturated fats, while limiting fruit. It also allows small amounts of dairy.[12]

The Paleolithic Diet is based on theories regarding our Paleolithic ancestors, as described in chapter 7. Proponents of this diet point out that our Paleolithic ancestors appear to have been hunter/gatherers much longer than they were farmers. The Paleolithic Period is believed to have spanned some two million years, while farming is believed to have started (in earnest) about 10,000 years ago. Therefore, it is reasonable to suggest our bodies are better adapted to eating flesh foods, vegetables, and fruit, as compared to grains, legumes, and dairy.[13,14,15]

Strong Points
- As with the previous diet, this one uses common foods that are fairly easy to get.
- Although you can prepare elaborate dishes, and be creative, meals can be very simple — meat and vegetables, with fruits and nuts as snacks or dessert.
- It discourages the use of salt, MSG, artificial sweeteners, processed meats, and factory-raised animals.
- It eliminates common allergens such as wheat, soy, peanuts, and dairy.

- Since some vegetables and virtually all fruit do not require cooking, the diet can include a large amount of raw food, including small amounts of raw animal products, such as sushi. In fact, some versions of this diet use significant amounts of raw meat.
- This diet is arguably the simplest and most "natural" of the low-carb diets, because, in its purest form, it consists essentially of meat, vegetables and fruit. In general, the diet emphasizes foods that have had a minimum amount of processing, and encourages organically-grown plant foods, grass-fed beef, wild-caught fish, and free-range poultry, as well as advocating sustainable agriculture.

Weak Points and Criticisms
- Most nutritional authorities consider 35% protein to be excessive. The modern Paleolithic Diet recommends that 50% of daily calories come from animal products. However, recent studies suggest that the proportion of animal products in the diets of our Paleolithic ancestors may have been considerably lower. Yes, they appear to have been hunter/gatherers for quite a long time, but it looks like they gathered more than they hunted.[16,17]
- The originator of this diet points out that humans have been cultivating grains and legumes for only 10,000 years or so, and therefore, he asserts that we have not had the time to biologically adapt to these foods. However, population studies suggest that some adaptation has occurred. For example, Northern Europeans seem to handle dairy better than Africans. Furthermore, recent analysis of Paleolithic fossils suggest that our ancestors started consuming starchy vegetables and even grains, long before they settled down into agricultural communities — at least 105,000 years ago.
- The diet of our Paleolithic ancestors was not necessarily the diet for optimum health; it was simply the diet that allowed them to survive and reproduce, even though their ancestral food (fruit) was no longer readily available. In other words, their diet may have changed, but their nutritional needs, according to some paleontologists, remained essentially the same as that of the anthropoid apes.[18,19]

My Opinion
As with the Weston A. Price Diet, the weak points and criticisms described above do not necessarily "debunk" the potential benefits. I would simply suggest

the individual be more flexible with the proportions of plant food to animal food, so as to suit personal needs.

I am inclined to think that many individuals on this diet would be better served if the proportion of animal food were more like 25%, rather than 50%, while still including generous servings of fruits and vegetables. This would actually be more consistent with the current thinking of paleontologists, as mentioned above. Better still, I think the ideal way to select food is to rely on personal experience and instinct, as do animals in the wild. In other words, if this dietary system "speaks" to you, just follow its basic guidelines (meat, fruit, vegetables), but pay attention to your inner signals, and adjust the proportion of plant to animal foods to fit your needs.

High-protein Low-carb Diets

Unlike other low-carb diets, this one is also low in fat. This is typically accomplished by using processed foods, such as soy powder, milk protein, and egg white.

Caloric Ratio: Carbs 5-30% Protein 30-60% Fat 20-30%

The purpose of the high protein intake is rapid weight loss. However, you pay the price in the form of deficiencies, tissue degeneration, and rapid aging of vital organs.[20] The fact that this diet relies on non-whole food (protein extracts) is reason enough for concern. The protein content may easily exceed 40% of daily calories, and can be as high as 60%. At such high levels, protein toxicity might actually be high enough to become noticeable as weakness, nausea, and diarrhea. This sort of diet, at best, should be done only for a limited time, and preferably under clinical supervision.

I first encountered protein toxicity early on in my practice as a chiropractor. One of my patients came in with a flare-up of low back pain, and also complained of nausea and generally not feeling well. When she mentioned having recently started a diet consisting of massive amounts of animal products and huge amounts of protein, I explained that such a diet can be stressful to the liver and kidneys, which would explain her symptoms, including the low back pain. I suggested that she simply reduce the animal products, and make room for a goodly amount of fruits and vegetables. She did so, and rapidly improved.

Reduced-protein Low-carb Diets

The high-protein diet, described above, has an extreme version of a feature that is shared by most low-carb diets — high protein levels. This feature has resulted in much of the criticism against these diets. Therefore, it was just a matter of time before some pioneering nutritional teachers came up with a reduced-protein version of the low-carb diet. This is accomplished by simply reducing the animal products and increasing plant foods, including carefully selected sources of plant-based fats.[21]

Caloric ratio: carbs 35% protein 15% fat 60%

The inclusion of more plant foods has the added advantage of providing more of the micronutrients that allow for the efficient elimination of toxins. However, since this sort of diet has not been around too long, we cannot really say anything definitive about it. Nonetheless, as with other diets, there have been enough reports of success to create a following, as well as to merit further investigation.[22]

The "Crossover" Diets

The Zone Diet

The Zone Diet is an example of a diet that attempts to be somewhat "neutral" or "balanced" regarding the source of calories. Its goal is to balance hormones to control hunger on fewer calories, while still getting the proper amount of micronutrients. Compared to the low-carb diets, the carbohydrate content is on the high side, consequently the fat is on the low side. The protein content is similar to what we see in most low-carb diets.

Caloric Ratio: Carbs 40% Protein 30% Fats 30%

Strong Points
- It is said to be effective for managing blood sugar and promoting weight loss.
- It is doable for the average person. For example, when eating at home, the ideal high-protein foods are chicken, turkey, salmon, sardines,

mackerel, and beans. To do this, add twice the amount of high-fiber veggies and whole grain products.

Weak Points and Criticisms
- Though the developer of The Zone Diet describes it as a moderate-carbohydrate, moderate-protein, moderate-fat diet, it has received the same criticism as other low carb diets — not enough carbohydrates and too much protein, resulting in deficiencies of vitamins, minerals, and loss of calcium.

The Gluten-free Diet

Gluten is a protein found in certain grains — wheat, barley, rye, and, to a lesser extent, oats. Many individuals are allergic to gluten. When the gluten sensitivity is severe enough, it is called celiac disease, which is characterized by destruction of the inner lining of the small intestine.

Strong Points
- Since this diet eliminates glutenous grains, it is ideal for individuals who have celiac disease, but can also be very helpful for many others whose health issues might stem from low-grade gluten sensitivity.
- Elimination of gluten is relatively easy for individuals who follow a low-carb diet. In fact, many of the reported benefits of low-carb diets are due to reduction or elimination of gluten.
- This diet is also doable for those on low-fat diets, simply by utilizing more fruit and non-glutenous grains, such as millet, rice, and amaranth, as well as starchy vegetables, such as potatoes, sweet potatoes, and winter squash.

Weak Points and Criticisms
The only disadvantage to this diet is that it necessitates the elimination of common foods that the individual may have previously depended on, as a matter convenience or as a matter of taste. Either way, the individual might have to go through a period of adjustment.

The Blood Type Diet

The Blood Type Diet is unique among the others, because it does not present a single formula for all humans. This diet, developed by Peter D'Adamo,

N.D., uses the ABO blood groups as the primary factor for determining the diet of an individual. Therefore, the percentage of carbohydrates, fats, and proteins can vary considerably from one individual to the next.

The dietary guidelines are based on the presence of chemicals in foods, called lectins. Different foods have different lectins. These lectins can react differently depending on the blood type of the individual. Based on these reactions, every food is categorized as being "beneficial," "neutral," or "avoid" for a given blood type.[23,24] Based on this distinction, the diet offers the following guidelines:

- If you have blood type "O," you are said to be relatively well-adapted to red meat and most vegetables and fruits, but should avoid dairy and most grains and legumes. The developer of the blood type diet suggests that the dietary preference of blood type "O" came about during the hunter/gatherer period of our ancestors.
- If you are blood type "A," you can chow down on virtually all grains, most legumes, and most types of vegetables and fruits, while exercising moderation with animal products, avoiding red meat altogether. Blood type A is said to be an adaptation to the development of agriculture that followed the hunter-gatherer period of our ancestors.
- Blood types "B" and "AB" are said to be sort of in between A and O.

Strong Points
- There are enough reported positive results from this diet that some naturopathic schools teach it in their programs.
- The diet encourages whole organic foods.

Weak Points and Criticisms
- Some critics claim the positive results from this diet are due to a general improvement in food quality, rather than blood type considerations.
- The theoretical basis for this diet, as presented by Dr. D'Adamo, has been widely criticized. Part of it has to do with Dr. D'Adamo's assertion that the blood types originated as a consequence of the changing diet of our ancestors, rather than simply suggesting that the evolution of the ABO blood groups in humans were *influenced* by diet.
- Though some correlations have been found between physiological tendencies and the ABO blood groups, they are not necessarily consistent with Dr. D'Adamo's dietary guidelines.

My Opinion

Some aspects of the theory behind the blood type diet do seem flawed. For example, the ABO blood groups exist in anthropoid apes.[25] However, "flawed" is not the same as totally wrong. Over the years, I have seen enough (potential) association between blood type and food reaction (in myself, as well as my students and patients) that I would not totally dismiss the entire concept. In other words, I have noted some patterns regarding the ABO blood types and diet, even if the patterns don't quite conform to Dr. D'Adamo's specifications. My observations include specific positive results that I would be hard-pressed to explain in terms of "general improvement" in food quality. Therefore, I suspect the blood type might, indeed, be a piece of the nutrition puzzle, even if it is not the most important piece, and even if Dr. D'Adamo's interpretation of it is in need of revision.

The South Beach Diet

The South Beach Diet was developed by Arthur Agatston, M.D. and Marie Almon, R.D. Dr. Agatston, a cardiologist, found some patients did not do well with the low-fat diets recommended for heart patients. This diet allows more carbohydrates than the other low-carb diets because one of its goals is to moderately reduce the overall fat in the diet. The diet uses lean meats, poultry, fish, nuts, and seeds as the major sources of protein and fat.

The calories lost from the reduction of total fat are replaced by whole-food sources of carbohydrates, such as fruits, vegetables, beans, and whole grains. The initial phase of the diet is strictly low-carb, but eventually whole-food carbohydrates are added and the fat and protein are proportionately reduced. The revised version of the Atkins Diet uses a similar strategy.

Caloric Ratio: Carbs 35-65% Protein 15-25% Fats 20-35%

Strong Points
- The diet eliminates refined carbohydrates, and features whole foods.
- As with the Paleo Diet, this one restricts trans-fats, and reduces saturated fats and omega-6 fats, replacing them with foods rich in omega-3 fats.
- This diet is flexible and allows for individuals who may prefer more or less animal based foods. Dr. Agatston even provides for a vegetarian version of the South Beach Diet.[26]

Weak Points and Criticism
- This diet relies heavily on the glycemic index, which, according to most dietitians and some nutrition authorities, has only limited value in predicting the effect of a food on overall blood sugar.
- Though the diet permits a substantial amount of plant foods, the initial phase of the diet excludes carbohydrate foods entirely, which results in rapid loss of water-weight and loss of minerals.

Though this diet has been described as a low-carb diet, Dr. Agatston does not particularly care for that label. He says that his diet is so flexible it would be inaccurate to call it "low-carb." I think he may have a point there. In one sense, this diet is like a bridge between the low-carb diets, described above, and the low-fat diets, described below.

Low-fat Diets

The low-fat diets are low in fat because they are high in carbohydrates. Most of these diets rely on starchy plant foods, such as grains, potatoes, and squash, for the bulk of daily calories. A few of them reduce the starchy foods and replace them with larger amounts of fruits and low-starch vegetables.

Caloric Ratio: Carbs 60-80% Protein 10-15% Fats 10-25%

Strong Points
- Low-fat diets greatly reduce or eliminate the over-consumption of factory-farmed animal products and the excessive consumption of protein, while guiding the individual to whole-foods sources of carbohydrates.
- These diets, when done properly, have proven to be very effective in reversing cardiovascular disease, diabetes mellitus, and obesity.

Weak Points and Criticisms
- This dietary approach, if not done properly, can result in the over-consumption of grains and refined sugar, leading to weight gain, blood sugar issues, and arthritis.[27]
- Low-fat diets tend to be mostly or completely vegetarian, and therefore have been associated with deficiencies in vitamin B_{12}, vitamin D, and long-chain omega-3 oils, such as EPA and DHA, all of which can

create neurological problems — as well as the same cardiovascular issues attributed to excessive protein and fat. For example, low levels of B_{12} can result in irreversible brain damage, as well as triggering high blood levels of homocysteine, which is associated with irritation of the inner lining of blood vessels that trigger vascular disease.
- Just as excessive amounts of fats have been associated with a number of toxicity issues, low levels of fat can produce various deficiencies by inhibiting the absorption of minerals and fat-soluble nutrients.

Regarding the fat, how low is too low? And how much does it vary from person to person? Only time will tell. In the meantime, the health seeking public might become confused by proponents of low-carb diets who claim that *everyone* can thrive on a diet that provides 50% (or more) of calories from fat, while the proponents of low-fat diets claim that the ideal amount *for everyone* is 10-20% (or less). Which end of the spectrum is best for you? You are the best judge of that, in my opinion.

Three well-known examples of low-fat diets are the Macrobiotic, Pritikin, and Ornish Diets.

The Macrobiotic Diet

Macrobiotics is basically a modification of the traditional Japanese diet, using an abundance of cooked grains (typically rice) to provide the bulk of the calories, as well as cooked vegetables, legumes, sea vegetation, and a moderate amount of fish and fermented products, such as miso. The diet has very little fruit. Onions and garlic are excluded because they are said to stimulate the appetite too much, and promote overeating. Nightshades (potatoes, tomatoes, peppers) are also excluded. The percentage of carbohydrates, fats, and proteins tends to be fairly close to the NIH guidelines, though the numbers can vary moderately.

Strong Points
- It uses mostly whole foods, avoids refined and highly processed wheat and sugar, and eliminates the over-consumption of animal products.
- It reportedly has been used to help with degenerative conditions such as cancer, heart disease, and arthritis.
- It can be done as a strictly plant-based diet or can include fish.
- In addition to the professed health benefits, the Macrobiotic Diet is economical, because grains and beans are both relatively inexpensive.

Weak Point and Criticisms
- It has been criticized for not having enough fresh fruit.
- The high-sodium, soy-based condiments tend to be addictive, making it difficult to restrict intake.

The Pritikin Diet

The Pritikin Diet was the first of the modern low-fat diets. It was created by Nathan Pritikin, and modified by his son, Robert Pritikin, M.D. It is based on grains, legumes, vegetables, and relatively small amounts of fruits. In this diet, fat and protein are each limited to about 10%. Animal products are allowed in small amounts.

As with the Atkins Diet, this one shows great short-term results. In this case, the diet has proven to be effective in reversing cardiovascular disease. In fact, the great results and the well-documented studies compelled the medical profession to finally acknowledge that there is, indeed, a connection between diet and cardiovascular disease. When Nathan Pritikin finally died (from a long-standing battle with leukemia), an autopsy was done, and revealed that his arteries were uncharacteristically clean and pliable for a 69 year old man.[28]

However, the long-term consumption of large amounts of grains has proven to be problematical for some individuals. There have been reports of higher incidences of arthritis and breast cancer.[29] These issues could possibly be related to a very high intake of soy and hybridized wheat, and the introduction of GMO wheat, corn, and soy.

The Ornish Diet

Created by Dean Ornish, M.D., this diet, like the Pritikin Diet, is based on grains, legumes, vegetables, and fruits. Fat is restricted to 10% or lower. A small amount of animal products are permitted.

Dr. Ornish developed this diet as part of a comprehensive system that includes exercise, yoga, meditation and support groups for patients that were diagnosed with cardiovascular disease.[29] The reversal of cardiovascular disease was so impressive that the program is now covered by many insurance companies.

Vegetarians and Vegans

Low-fat diets are either mostly or totally plant-based. The term "vegetarian" is often loosely applied to describe anyone who does not consume animal flesh, but might still eat some dairy and eggs. **The Vegan Diet** is a version of vegetarianism that excludes all foods derived from animals. The term "ethical vegan" is applied to individuals motivated by humane, spiritual, or environmental reasons. Such individuals exclude clothing or any other personal items using animal products or animal testing.

Vegetarianism, including ethical veganism, is not new. Abstinence from animal flesh is common in many of the religions of the world, especially in Asian countries. In ancient Greece, the philosophical order founded by Pythagoras included a vegetarian diet for both health and spiritual reasons. In fact, throughout history in the West, right up to the latter 19th century, those who followed a vegetarian diet were called "Pythagorians."[30]

Strong Points

- An abundance of whole plant foods provides a lot of fiber, which is essential for a clean and healthy digestive tract.
- Plant foods provide most of the needed minerals, vitamins, and all the phytonutrients needed to maintain a healthy body.
- Plant foods tend to leave less toxic residue than animal products.
- Numerous studies associate traditional plant-based diets with longevity.[31]

Weak Points and Criticisms

- Modern vegetarians and vegans often over-consume grains and highly processed soy products, both of which tend to produce allergic reactions.
- Both grains and soy can be addictive. Grains, especially wheat, contain opiates. Soy, especially highly processed soy protein, has high levels of glutamates, which combines with the salt that is usually added, to form monosodium glutamate, which is also addictive.
- Although the traditional cultures that have been reported to enjoy above-average health and longevity do eat a predominantly plant-based diet, they also typically include small to moderate amounts of meat, dairy, or eggs (1-10% of calories). I find it interesting that the amount of animal products in these traditional diets is similar to what we encounter in the diet of chimpanzees in the wild. However, vegan authors have a tendency to use these findings to justify the total elimination of animal products.

How important is that small amount of animal-based food? There is currently no clear answer to this question; therefore, we cannot arbitrarily dismiss it as unimportant. Even when the diet is supplemented with vitamin B_{12} and omega-3 oils, there is still a real possibility that other important factors are provided by those small amounts of animal products — at least in some individuals. Granted, recent studies on modern vegan communities do show some positive results, but these must be considered preliminary.[32]

- Though modern vegetarian diets are typically designed to be low-fat, this is often not the case in actual practice. It is tempting and easy to add substantial amounts of fatty foods on top of the already carbohydrate-rich meals. It is easy to slather on enough butter or margarine, pour on oil, and munch on enough walnuts to turn the supposedly low-fat diet into a fatty feast. Some vegetarians unknowingly get 30-40% calories from fat, while also consuming substantial amounts of carbohydrates, and then wonder why they gain weight on their "low-fat" diet. As previously stated, when carbohydrates and fats are both present in significant amounts, they tend to "clash," resulting in indigestion, blood sugar issues, candida overgrowth, and overeating.

Not surprisingly, vegetarian diets that have been used effectively for weight loss, diabetes, and cardiovascular health are careful to keep the fat portion of the diet down in the range of 10-20% of daily calories. Dr. Joel Fuhrman's "Eat to Live Diet" goes one step further by advising the individual to also limit the amounts of calorically dense carbohydrates, favoring instead foods that pack more vitamins, minerals, and phytonutrients.

Dr. Fuhrman's Eat-to-Live Diet

Compared to other vegan diets, this one is atypical, because it does not rely on large amounts of starchy foods. As you may recall from chapter 7, the fundamental anatomy and physiology of humans is basically the same as other primates. In recognition of this, the Eat-to-Live Diet encourages us to eat an abundance of fresh fruits and vegetables.

This diet is on the low-fat side, though not as low as the other vegan diets. It puts less emphasis on keeping the fat low, and more emphasis on the quality of the food. In so doing, this diet softens the low-carb vs. low-fat debate, and instead reminds us to make sure we get our vitamins, mineral and phytonutrients.

Caloric Ratio: Carbs 60-70% Protein 10-17% Fats 15-30%

A typical day on the Eat-to-Live Diet features about one pound of raw vegetables, one pound of cooked vegetables, and at least four servings of fresh fruit. The higher levels of fruits and vegetables reflect a proportionate reduction in cooked grains and starchy vegetables.

Nuts, seeds, avocados, and tofu are limited to a few ounces per day. Fruit juice, dried fruit, and animal products are avoided. However, this diet does provide options for individuals who want to use small amounts of animal products. Here again, Dr. Fuhrman softens the vegan vs. omnivore argument, because it distracts us from the fact that a diet that is calorically dominated by either meat or starchy foods is likely to produce long-term problems, related to toxicity and deficiency — because both of these food groups, in large amounts, crowd out the fresh fruits and vegetables that provide the health promoting vitamins, minerals, phytonutrients, and fiber.

Summary of Low-carb and Low-fat Diets

What We Know
- Both types of diets, done properly, have yielded good results in the form of better digestion, weight loss, and improved blood sugar.
- Low-fat diets have proven to be especially effective in reversing cardiovascular disease.
- Low-carb diets show promise in helping individuals with certain neurological disorders, such as Parkinson's disease and epilepsy. Done properly, they provide an alternative to individuals who, for one reason or another, do not respond well to a low-fat diet.
- In both systems, the benefits seem to be partially due to the practice of avoiding the mixing of large amounts of high-carb foods with large amounts of high-fat foods.
- In both systems, the benefits seem to be partially due to the elimination of refined and heavily processed food, favoring whole foods that provide an abundance of vitamins, minerals, and phytonutrients, and proper balance of omega 3 and omega 6 oils.
- Though many individuals get noticeable benefits from staying in their ideal caloric zone, the need to do so seems less critical as we improve food quality – clean whole foods, rich in micronutrients. In other words, your zone becomes effectively "wider" as you improve food quality.

What We Don't Know
- There is a need for more data on the difference between animal-based and plant-based low-carb diets.
- A recurring issue that is shared by both low-carb and low-fat diets is the emergence of long-term toxicity or deficiency symptoms, which apparently were not anticipated by the creators of the diets.
- There is a lack of data on individual differences. Some individuals might do well in the low-carb zone, while others might do better in the low-fat zone. Some individuals may have a "wide" zone, while others might have a "narrow" zone. Furthermore, an individual's ideal zone may very well change somewhat with the seasons of the year, as well as the seasons of his or her life.

Where Is *My* Zone?

In the presence of so many unknowns and varying opinions, here are three simple guidelines that can help you make sense of things:
- Relax, and trust your judgment.
- It's okay to change your mind.
- Choices are easier when you remember that you choose only for yourself.

In other words, after you learn what the authorities have to say, trust your own discernment and personal experience regarding what *you* need to eat. For example, some authors say 10% fat is sufficient, others say 15-30%, others say 40-60%. Which is right for you? In my opinion, *You* are ultimately the best judge of that.

The really good news is that healthy eating becomes simpler as you approach your ideal diet. As suggested earlier, if you use the caloric map properly, you can eventually put it away. Also, the need to "stay in your zone" seems less critical as you increase your consumption of clean whole foods that provide an abundance of micronutrients. In fact, when eating is restored to the purely instinctual act that it was intended to be, you can pretty much forget where your caloric zone is, because your body remembers, and will guide you accordingly.

In the meantime, as you continue your nutritional exploration, regardless of how promising a new diet looks, remember to see it for what it really is — an experiment.

Raw Food Diets

The word "experiment" is certainly a proper one to describe a diet consisting mostly or entirely of raw foods. Most of the traditional diets throughout the world are dominated by cooked food — and have been for thousands of years. Nonetheless, the current raw food diets merit close inspection for the following reasons:

- Widespread reports suggest that the right kind of raw diet can help reverse serious diseases, such as inoperable cancer and other forms of degeneration.
- In recent years, the raw diets have seen a rise in popularity, and have become a thriving business, with much fanfare, pontification, and showmanship, featuring countless books, websites, radio shows, seminars, and festivals.
- The potential benefits and emerging public interest associated with this sort of diet seem to have attracted promoters who are willing to sacrifice truth and integrity for the sake of appearance and financial success. Such behavior has muddied the waters regarding the benefits and limitations of eating raw.

The Need for Candor

As with cooked food diets, there has been a tendency among the raw food teachers to highlight the successes, while downplaying the challenges. The success stories might be useful and even inspiring, but the rough spots encountered along the way are equally important for individuals who seriously want to explore a particular diet. It is unfortunate that such information is often censored.

Hopefully, as more health-seeking individuals take the time to educate themselves, the showmanship and deception will fall away. An educated consumer will also create an opening for sincere teachers who have enough respect for the truth to avoid the temptation to censor or distort information.

The History of Raw Eating

The modern raw food movement began quietly in the early 20th century through the work of several pioneers who were attempting to treat conditions that did not respond well to conventional medicine.[33,34] The one pioneer that seems to have galvanized the modern raw food movement was A.T. Hovannessian.[35] He published a book called *Raw Eating* in 1960.

Prior to Hovannessian's work, raw food was used mostly by a few maverick medical doctors and other health practitioners, who were basically trying to follow the advice of Hippocrates, the recognized father of medicine, who said "Let food be your medicine, and medicine your food." However, after successfully applying their raw-food therapies, these pioneers typically guided their patients to adapt what was considered a healthy cooked-food diet.

Hovanessian went one step further. He declared, "Natural foodstuffs must not be utilized by doctors as merely temporary therapeutic means. They must be declared the only diet suitable for human beings."[36]

Whether or not we agree with Hovannessian's assertion, the use of raw food continues to grow in popularity. It also has some points of controversy. Therefore, let us now look at the advantages and disadvantages of cooked and raw food.

Advantages of Cooking
- Neutralizes toxins and antinutrients.
- Releases some nutrients (especially minerals) locked up in the plant fiber.
- Warms and softens food for easier digestion.
- Effectively increases the caloric value of the food.
- Allows us to utilize food sources, such as dry beans and grains, which are otherwise unavailable.
- Sterilizes food, allowing us to safely consume animal products.

Disadvantages of Cooking
- Cooking destroys some vitamins, phytonutrients, and all enzymes.
- Cooking oxidizes fats, making them toxic.
- Cooking carbohydrates produces carcinogenic substances called acrylamides.
- Cooking proteins at high temperatures produces protein-carbohydrate complexes that promote low-grade inflammation, degeneration, and aging of tissues.
- Cooking might render some of the protein unavailable. The heat either denatures the protein (making it less digestible) or destroys amino acids. For example, cooking releases the sulfur from some amino acids. The sulfur becomes sulfuric acid, which has a strong acidifying influence.

Advantages of Raw

The absence of cooked food means the body does not have to expend energy and resources to make the extra enzymes needed for digestion and cleanup.

Diets rich in raw fruits and vegetables have been shown to protect against cancer. For example, some of the nutrients in raw vegetables have been shown to facilitate removal of carcinogens and promote DNA repair.[37]

- Delicate vitamins, phytonutrients, and enzyme are preserved. The latter is actually a point of controversy. See Appendix B for a full discussion on this topic.
- Some studies, such as Kirlian photography, have revealed that foods have electromagnetic qualities that seem to be strongest in freshly picked raw fruits and vegetables, especially those that receive the most sunlight, such as tropical fruit. However, it is still not clear how the stronger energy field of raw food benefits the individual eating the food.

Disadvantages of Raw

- When raw foods are improperly grown and stored, they can harbor pathogens.
- Since most of our readily available foods are cooked, the diet might be logistically difficult.
- Calorie for calorie, fresh fruits and vegetables tend to be more expensive than grains, potatoes, and beans.
- Since individuals who eat this way are in the minority, the diet might be socially stressful.
- Even if a 100% raw diet is doable from a logistical standpoint, it may still not be beneficial for a given individual due to the need for nutrients in concentrations that are unavailable or difficult to get in a totally raw vegan diet.

Navigating through the Raw Food World

Raw diets are usually vegan, but when animal products are present, they are typically in very small amounts. Beyond that, the world of raw diets, interestingly enough, has a landscape that mirrors that of cooked food diets. For example, we see two major versions of raw diets — low-fruit and a high-fruit, which parallel the low-carb and low-fat diets, previously discussed. Furthermore, as with the cooked food diets, there is much debate and sometimes conflict among the proponents of these two raw systems.

Low-fruit Raw

The low-fruit raw diets are usually, but not necessarily, low-carb, meaning the percentage of calories derived from carbohydrates tends to be below the NIH recommendations (chapter 8). The carbohydrates are on the low side because fruit is restricted, and the usual cooked high-carb foods (grains, beans, and starchy vegetables) have been eliminated. Such a diet usually provides the bulk of calories (40-70%) from fatty foods — nuts, seeds, avocados, coconuts, and extracted oils.

As with the cooked low-carb diets, the advocates of the low-fruit raw diets believe that larger amounts of fat is safe and healthy if it is of a high quality. In this case, fats have not been heated above physiological temperatures, making them more user-friendly. This is a valid point, because heating does oxidize fats, especially polyunsaturated oils, which can be a major source of toxicity, if the fats are consumed in large amounts.

Strong Points

- Proponents of the low-fruit raw diets would agree that it is beneficial to limit the fat intake (somewhat). They might do this by moderately increasing fresh fruit, as well as including generous amounts of freshly squeezed vegetable juices and a variety of soaked and sprouted seeds that are lower in fat (millet, quinoa, oats, buckwheat. amaranth, alfalfa).
- By using the above strategy, dietary fat can be reduced to the point that the diet is no longer "low-carb," while still keeping the fruit on the low side. For example, Max Gerson, one of the early pioneers in the therapeutic use of raw food, gave his cancer patients large amounts of freshly squeezed vegetable juice. Fruit was also considered beneficial, but it was kept moderate, so as to make room for large amounts of vegetables and their juices. He was also adamant about keeping the fat very low, because he said most fatty foods promote tumor growth.
- Another way that raw diets reduce the fat is by simply restricting total calories. In other words, the individual simply "under eats." Reducing calories, while still supplying the body with an abundance of vitamins, minerals, and phytonutrients has proven to be an effective strategy for promoting deep cleansing and healing. In fact, this is precisely the sort of program that has given the raw diet a reputation for helping reverse serious diseases.

Weak Points and Criticisms
- The low-calorie and high-micronutrient approach, though potentially very effective as a therapeutic measure, must eventually give way to a maintenance diet that provides adequate calories to maintain weight. Since fruit is restricted, the only other realistic raw alternative is to substantially increase fat consumption. Doing this for a long time has proven to be problematical for many individuals.
- The question is, how much fat is too much? And how much does it vary from person to person? Unfortunately, the answer is not any clearer for raw food than it is for cooked. Some individuals seem to do well with higher levels of fat; others do not.
- To complicate matters, the high-fat raw foods used in this sort of diet are often not merely consumed in their pristine form, or in simple combinations, but rather are incorporated into complex recipes (that often include added salt and extracted oils), and involve considerable mixing, blending, and exposure to hot air in a dehydrator, which subject the food to oxidation and loss of nutrients. In so doing, we lose much of the cleaning and healing virtues ascribed to raw food. These complex high-fat foods include the raw analogues of pizza, lasagna, tacos, dumplings, cheesecake, and apple pie. They are often quite delicious, but are also the antithesis of the simple raw foods used by the early pioneers to successfully treat serious degenerative diseases.
- There has been a tendency among some of the promoters of these diets to be somewhat "fruit-phobic." As with the promoters of the cooked low-carb diets, they warn the public about eating more than a small amount of fruit. Granted, some individuals do have issues that necessitate the restriction of fruit, as described below, but this should not be used as justification to vilify fruit as food.

High-fruit Raw

This version of the raw diet tends to be very low in fat (10% or lower is common), though some individuals do allow for moderately higher levels. As with the cooked low-fat diets, this diet provides the bulk of daily calories from carbohydrates. In this case, the carbohydrates come mostly from fresh fruit. Though fruit is substantially lower in calories than grains and starchy vegetables, it can still meet our caloric needs — we just have to eat more of it. In addition to fruit, this diet usually includes substantial amounts of vegetables and small amounts of high-fat foods, such as nuts, seeds, and avocados.

Strong Points
- This diet, by its very nature, is cleansing for the body, because fruit has a high water content, lots of fiber, and the least amount of toxic residue of all food groups. Individuals on this diet often report a decrease of body odor, and they often claim, "My poop doesn't stink anymore."
- Regarding blood sugar, according to the proponents of this diet, when the body has been allowed to cleanse and balance itself, fresh fruits generally do not contribute to blood sugar problems or yeast overgrowth. The major cause of blood sugar problems and candida is said to be high levels of fat, and other stressors, that inhibit the body's ability to absorb and utilize sugars.[38]
- The macronutrients in fruit are largely predigested, allowing the body to conserve energy, which is then available for other purposes, such as deeper cleansing and regeneration.
- Individuals on this diet often report steady energy, with no fluctuation or fatigue. This might be partially due to the energy conserved from the ease of digestion and cleanup. In addition, most of the common fruits contain malic acid, which, among its other benefits, is also burned for energy more efficiently than the sugars. For this reason, malic acid is often used to help individuals with chronic fatigue syndrome and fibromyalgia. Fruits highest in malic acid include apples, pears, peaches, pineapples, grapes, cherries, and raspberries.

Weak Points and Criticisms
- Proponents of this diet sometimes point out that humans evolved in the tropics, and are therefore adapted to eat lots of fruit. However, most modern humans do not live in the tropics. In fact, the majority of humans come from a lineage of hundreds or even thousands of generations of ancestors living in temperate or cold climates.
- Calorie for calorie, fruit tends to be more expensive than grains, beans, and potatoes.
- Though large amounts of fruit sugars can be utilized more efficiently when dietary fat is reduced, this does not mean a given individual can consume fruit in massive quantities. Some individuals might have liver issues that impede the proper utilization of the fructose found in fruit. For example, large amounts of fructose can possibly result in elevated triglycerides and uric acid.
- The protein content of this diet might be too low for some individuals.

- Deficiency in omega-3 fats may occur.
- If the overall fat content is *too* low, it could hinder the absorption of some minerals and fat-soluble vitamins.
- Mineral deficiencies, such as zinc or selenium, may occur if the individual eats too much fruit and not enough vegetables.
- If this diet is practiced in a strictly vegan manner, which is usually the case, it could produce a deficiency of vitamin B_{12} as well as low levels of the amino acids, cysteine and methionine. These issues can result in elevated blood levels of homocysteine, which irritates the inner lining of blood vessels, and is proving to be a more accurate predictor of cardiovascular disease than high cholesterol levels.
- In other words, the main issue with this sort of diet is not toxicity, but deficiency — the opposite of what we usually see with other diets.

The 80/10/10 Diet, is a popular version of the high-fruit and low-fat approach.[39] Here are the essential features of this diet:

- At least 80% of the daily calories come from carbohydrates. No more than 10% of calories come from protein — preferably lower. No more than 10% of calories come from fat — preferably lower.
- By the numbers, this diet is basically a fruitarian version of the cooked low-fat diets developed by Pritikin, Ornish, and others. The main difference is the source of calories — coming mostly from fresh fruit, instead of grains and starchy vegetables.
- In addition to fruits and vegetables, the diet allows 1-2 ounces of nuts and seeds or an avocado, a few times a week.
- Totally raw is recommended, but not required.

My opinion: 10% fat is accepted by most of the other vegan authors, and seems to work well for many individuals. However, *less* than 10% is another matter. In fact, Dr. Graham has stated that 5% fat is acceptable. 5% fat means that you essentially eat fruits and vegetables, and nothing else. Some individuals claim to thrive on this very low fat level, but that certainly does not mean that everyone can.

Opinions do vary widely on the fat question, and, unfortunately, the various authors tend to present their case with a high degree of certainty that is often unjustified by the available evidence, as well as failing to allow for individual differences. The potential benefits of this diet certainly make it worthy of consideration, but it should be approached with caution, if it is radically different from your usual way of eating. Again, any new diet that you try should be seen for what it really is — a personal experiment.

A Closer Look at Fruit

Fruit is enjoying a rise in popularity. More books (such as this one) are endorsing the eating of fruit. More nutritional authors are emerging who call themselves fruitarians or *frugavores*. For these reasons, as well as the potential issues that can arise for some individuals, let us take a closer look at a fruit.

One point of confusion about the high-fruit diet starts with the term, "Fruitarian," which like "vegetarian," has no strict definition. The term is often used to describe someone who gets the bulk of daily calories (roughly 75%) or more from fruit. For the sake of simplicity, I will use this unofficial definition.

A second point of confusion is the assumption that a fruitarian diet must necessarily be very low in fat. It usually is, but some individuals who call themselves fruitarians do eat fat in amounts well above 10%, even though the bulk of calories still come from the carbs in fruit.

Neither does the fruitarian diet have to be totally raw. Neither does it have to totally exclude animal products. Cooked or non-vegan foods, when present, typically consist of steamed vegetables, maybe small amounts of cooked grains and beans, or small amounts of raw goats milk, eggs, and flesh foods, such as fish.

In other words, there is quite a bit of diversity among so-called fruitarians. The only unifying feature is the use of fruit as the primary source of calories. However, even here, we see some disagreement on the semantics. Some individuals prefer the term "frugavore" to describe someone who gets the bulk of calories from fruit, while reserving the term "fruitarian" for those who eat *only* fruit.

Return of the Primate Diet

I guess it was inevitable that humans would eventually rediscover a diet resembling that of other primates. In addition to the potential health benefits, it has the romantic appeal of "returning to the garden." However, we should keep in mind that some anthropoid apes do eat small amounts of animal food. Even the primates that do not intentionally consume animal flesh probably ingest aphids and other tiny creatures without even trying. In contrast, humans who favor this way of eating typically follow a vegan diet, eating fruits and vegetables that have been washed clean of dirt and bugs.

By totally veganizing and sanitizing the primate diet, some long-term deficiencies could conceivably arise. This, in my opinion, is an important point to consider, one that is often overlooked by raw-food enthusiasts.

As mentioned above, critics of this sort of diet claim that large amounts of fruits are not an ideal source of calories, because the high levels of simple sugars and inadequate levels of protein, fats, and other nutrients. Proponents of this diet respond by suggesting that the need for more of some nutrients is due to the body being clogged with fat and other undigested debris and metabolic toxins, which compromise digestion and absorption. Also, they point out that the amount of fruit can be adjusted to suit individual needs, by simply including more vegetables, which would also moderately increase the protein and fat content. In a similar manner, fatty foods, such as avocados, nuts, seeds, and coconuts can be modestly increased.

Another potential issue is fructose, which, on average, makes up about half the sugars in fruit. Some studies have indicated that high levels of fructose might produce elevated uric acid and triglycerides. The latter could contribute to a fatty liver. Proponents of the high-fruit diet respond by pointing out that such studies are typically not done with fresh fruit, but refined fructose, as in high fructose corn syrup.[40] They also point out that such studies are typically done on individuals who were also eating substantial amounts of the usual cooked grains and animal products, not on individuals eating a high-fruit diet that was free of the usual cooked foods. They claim that the elimination of these potential stressors will allow the body to handle fruit sugars with more ease and grace. However, there have currently been no formal studies to substantial these claims.

How Much Fruit Is Right for Me?

Beyond all other points of disagreement, the real question is, how do you know if eating substantial amounts of fruit is right for *you*?

First of all, if the idea of eating a lot of fruit does not appeal to you, the answer is probably no. On the other hand, if you are curious enough to check it out, here is how you might begin: Gradually increase your fruit consumption (as described at the end of this chapter), and see how you feel. If you need further confirmation, check the pH of your urine with strips of pH paper. If your urine pH does not become more acidic, it suggests that your liver is processing the fructose very nicely. If your urine becomes more acidic, it suggests that your liver's capacity to process fructose might be compromised. If you need even more confirmation, you can check your blood sugar and triglycerides.

If all subjective and objective signs remain good, there really is no logical reason to stop yourself. You can just continue to gradually increase your fruit consumption to the level that feels right to you.

Can I Eat *Just* fruit?

The 100% Fruit Diet is not recommended by most nutritional authors, due to the low levels of protein, fats, and possibly minerals. Over all, sweet fruits have a caloric ratio that looks like this: Carbs 92%, protein 4%, fat 4%.

These levels of fat and protein are lower than those of any of the other food groups. As usual, protein gets most of the attention. And, indeed, in this case, we can legitimately question if the protein will be adequate for a given individual. However, the very low levels of fat are, at least, equally important. Specifically, there have been reports of mental and emotional instability and even deaths on such a diet. The low fat content is of special concern for young children, because their fat requirements are higher than adults.

Some strict fruitarians resolve the fat issue by simply including a generous amount of fatty fruits, such as avocados, which can easily raise the fat content from 4% to about 25% or higher.[41] Another strategy is to include more berries, since they tend to have twice the fat and protein of other fruits.

Also, individuals who claim to thrive for years on just fruit, do not just eat sweet fruit, but include non-sweet botanical fruits, such as cucumbers, bell peppers, tomatoes, and zucchini, all of which have a nutritional profile more closely resembling leafy vegetables. Using these strategies, the 100% fruit diet can easily have a caloric ratio recommended by most vegan authors — about 80/10/10!

Zucchini and Friends

Whether or not you have visions of becoming a fruitarian, the non-sweet botanical fruits have many blessings to offer. In one sense, they combine some of the benefits of the sweet fruits and green leafy vegetables. As with most sweet fruit, the non-sweet fruits, such as tomatoes, bell peppers, cucumbers, zucchini, and yellow summer squash, are compact, can be eaten raw, are portable, easy to store, and have a longer shelf life than leafy green vegetables. On the other hand, like leafy greens, these same non-sweet fruits are very low in calories and relatively high in vitamins, minerals, and phytonutrients, as well as offering moderately higher levels of protein and fat, compared to sweet fruits. For example, baby zucchini provides 31% of calories from protein and 17% from fat. In addition, the amino acid profile of zucchini resembles that of eggs, which are considered to be the standard in protein quality.

> Since all of the non-sweet fruits have a firmer texture than leafy greens, they can be cut up into bite-size pieces and combined with various sweet or savory dips or patés. Zucchini also have a texture that offers an interesting option in terms of food preparation. Zucchini can be processed through a spiralizer, which converts the fruit into a bunch of spaghetti-like strands. The zucchini pasta can then be topped with raw or cooked tomato sauce, to make a surprisingly delicious alternative to the usual high-starch spaghetti meal. Instead of tomato sauce, other toppings can be used, such as a lemon and tahini sauce, to make a delightful dish of sesame noodles. To create a texture that is closer to regular spaghetti, the zucchini pasta can be lightly steamed.

In her book, *Fruitarianism, The Path to Paradise*, Anne Osborne describes her experience of 17 years (21 years, as of this writing) of excellent health and fitness on a low-fat 100% fruit diet.[42] However, she does not claim that everyone can succeed on the diet she follows. She also explains the two major reasons why many individuals are unable to sustain a long-term 100% fruit diet:

- **Preparation.** The body needs time to cleanse and reset itself so that it is capable of extracting sufficient nutrients from fruit alone. Like other fruitarian authors, Osborne suggests that once the body has had sufficient time to adapt, the individual absorbs and utilizes the nutrients in fruit more efficiently.
- **Fruit quality.** Conventionally grown fruit usually lacks the nutritional profile necessary to sustain optimum health because of poor soil quality and the common practice of picking fruit before it is ripe. For example, by picking fruit prematurely, the mineral content will be lower, because as the fruit ripens, the higher sugar levels draw in minerals from the soil.

However, even if the two explanations given above prove to have merit, they should not be taken as a green light to jump into a 100% fruit diet, or even a mostly-fruit diet. On the contrary, the two challenges described by Osborne remind us that such a diet should be approached with caution and care by those used to eating the usual diet dominated by cooked grains or meat. This is especially true for individuals living in a cooler climate, where fresh tree-ripened fruit are more difficult to get.

Mostly Raw Diets

There are raw dietary systems that allow for modest amounts of selected cooked foods. The inclusion of cooked food allows the individual to get ample amounts of calories, protein, and fat without relying too heavily on high-fat raw foods, or large amounts of fruit. For example:

- The **Hallelujah Diet** allows for 15% cooked food.
- The **Hippocrates Diet** advocates raw on most days, with an occasional meal that includes certain cooked foods, such as grains or squash.
- The **Gerson Diet** uses raw fruits and vegetables and substantial amounts of amounts of freshly squeezed vegetable juice — as much as 15-20 pounds per day of juices, fruits, and vegetables to help individuals with cancer and other degenerative diseases. How do you get people to drink that much juice? It is simple; these individuals are motivated because they have life-threatening diseases. Since Dr. Gerson's research suggested that fatty foods tend to promote tumor growth, he usually excluded such foods. With fat restricted, the caloric needs are met by allowing a moderate amount of cooked plant-food in the evening meal.

The Best of Both Worlds

The question, "Should I cook or not cook?" might best be answered with the following rule of thumb: *Eat raw when you can, and cook food when you need to.* Beyond that, here are some simple guidelines to get the most benefit from cooked and raw foods, while minimizing the disadvantages of both.

Clean Cooking

- The production of toxins and destruction of nutrients through cooking tend to increase with higher temperature and longer cooking time. This can obviously be minimized by favoring shorter cooking time and lower temperature. Steaming and boiling are cleaner than broiling and frying.
- The known toxins produced by cooking come from the degradation of calorically dense foods, such as grains, starchy vegetables, nuts, seeds, and animal products. In contrast, the toxic residue produced by cooking beans or steaming vegetables is actually quite small. Steamed broccoli is a lot cleaner than French fries. Chicken soup made from free-range chicken, including the bones and organ meat, and mixed with a goodly amount of vegetables, makes a cleaner and more nutritious meal than batter-dipped mystery nuggets, deep fried in partially hydrogenated oil.

The Best of Raw

The main benefits of cooking are the warming and softening of food and the release of nutrients from the plant fiber. Here are several simple ways of regaining some of the benefits of cooking, even with raw foods:

- Do not eat raw fruits and vegetables straight out of the refrigerator, but rather allow them to warm up to room temperature, or find ways to gently warm them so as to be close (or to slightly above) body temperature.
- Favor fruits that are naturally soft. Such fruits tend to be readily available — strawberries, blackberries, blue berries, raspberries, peaches, mangos, papaya, bananas, figs, grapes, etc. Likewise, favor young tender greens, which have softer fiber than the mature plants.
- Processing fruits and vegetables quickly in a powerful blender breaks up fiber and liberates nutrients, similar to cooking, but with much less loss of nutrients through prolonged exposure to high heat.
- You can use warm or even hot water (not hot enough to burn your skin) to blend raw food. In fact, by using herbs and spices, you can make a savory and delicious vegetable soup or stew, which is hot enough to make a comforting and satisfying wintertime meal, but still raw.
- In the winter, I sometimes have a quick banana smoothie, consisting entirely of bananas blended in enough warm water to make a thick and surprisingly delicious "milk shake." Naturally, other fruits may be added for variety of textures and flavors. Raw vegetables can also be added. For example, I sometimes enjoy a warm smoothie made of bananas and romaine lettuce. Or, I throw in some carob powder to make a "chocolate milk shake."
- Dates, carob powder, and coconut meat can be blended in hot water to make a creamy and surprisingly delicious hot "chocolate."
- Raw apple sauce is another wintertime food I enjoy. First, I might warm up 2-4 apples through various means, such as placing them in a warm water bath. Then I run them through a powerful blender until they become warm applesauce. I sometimes add a dash of cinnamon and ginger.
- Another one of my wintertime treats is my version of figgy pudding, consisting entirely of dried figs blended in hot water (not too hot). The more powerful blenders reduce the figs to a delightfully smooth and creamy consistency. With the less powerful blenders, you can first soak the figs in warm water for a few hours, but the pudding will probably still come out sort of chunky after blending. Smooth or chunky, both are delicious.

Cleaning Up Your Diet

In summary, each of the diets described in this chapter has its own plan for delivering all the needed nutrients to the body. However, as explained in chapter 4, the ease of digestion and cleanup that follow the meal are of equal importance to the actual nutrient content. For this reason, the lessons learned from the high-fruit diet can be of value for everyone, regardless of which dietary system you happen to favor.

Building-foods and Cleansing-foods Revisited

As explained in chapter 4, high-calorie foods, such as grains, beans, nuts, seeds, and animal products, are called building-foods, because they provide the fuel and building materials to build and run the body. On the other hand, fruits and vegetables are called cleansing-foods, because they are relatively low in calories, but high in water, fiber, vitamins, minerals, and phytonutrients, all of which promote cleansing.

As you may recall, the primary cause of the major degenerative diseases is too much of the building-foods (too many calories), and not enough of the cleansing-foods. In fact, the *excess* of calorie-dense foods is the most obvious cause of the diseases of civilization. The body simply does not have the opportunity to adequately cleanse itself.

The idea of giving strong attention to ease of digestion and cleansing is not new. In ancient Greece, Hippocrates said, "Let food be your medicine, and medicine your food." What foods was he referring to? Fruits and vegetables — mostly raw! More recently, Natural Hygiene has championed the cleansing side of eating.

Natural Hygiene

Natural Hygiene, founded in the United States in the early 1800s, is not a diet, per se. It is an integrated system of healing and healthy living.[43] In addressing health challenges, Natural Hygiene refrains from using drugs, herbal remedies, or any invasive therapeutic procedure, but rather engages the body's own self-healing capacity, through fasting, rest, proper exercise, clean water, clean air, and sunshine. Seems very simple, but it can be surprisingly difficult to implement, because we have been conditioned to go for remedies that produce fast results. Herbert Shelton, one of prominent Natural Hygienists in the mid 20th century said, "One of the hardest things to do is nothing."

To underscore what Hippocrates said about food and medicine, Natural Hygiene teaches that the same foods that maintain the body in a healthy state can also be used to allow for the healing of pathological conditions. Regarding everyday eating, Natural Hygiene favors a simple diet consisting of fresh fruits and vegetables as the main features. Some Natural Hygiene authors recommend a totally raw diet; others use moderate amounts of cooked food. Some are strict vegans; others use modest amounts of animal products.

Paradoxically, Natural Hygiene is not very well-known in the United States, but has gained more popularity in other countries, especially in the United Kingdom and Eastern Europe, where it became part of the natural health movement in the early 20th century — which eventually gave rise to the modern raw food movement.

Any given dietary system can potentially become more sustainable by simply including the common sense principles promoted by Natural Hygiene, such as the simple practice of occasionally letting the body rest from the usual foods.

Granted, a diet consisting of mostly or totally raw fruits and vegetables is radically different from the everyday eating habits of most modern humans. Though it is precisely what Hippocrates recommended some 2,500 years ago, most individual living on Planet Earth right now would find it impractical for one reason or another. Nonetheless, the overall nutritional profile of fruit, along with its ease of digestion and low toxic residue, provide us with an option that, until recently, has been mostly overlooked or actively dismissed by other mainstream dietary systems: the use of fruit as a staple food.

Fruit as a Staple Food

Using fruit as a staple food does not necessarily mean you become a fruitarian. It simply means that fruit is consumed in quantities that make a significant contribution to the fulfillment of our daily caloric needs. By the numbers, if we consume enough fresh fruit to provide 10% of daily calories, we could legitimately say that fruit is being used as a staple food.

The value of using fruit as staple food is simply that it makes us less dependent on the other more concentrated sources of calories, most notably grains and animal products, which, by their very nature, are more difficult to digest and leave a higher toxic residue. By thus reducing the burden on the body, fruit can make any diet cleaner and more sustainable. In fact, this is precisely what some diets have done. For example, the Pritikin Diet used to severely restricted fruit, and the original Atkins Diet banned it altogether. Both diets eventually encountered difficulties associated with toxicity. Both diets responded by allowing for more fruit.

What does 10% fruit look like? Based on the standard 2,000-calorie diet, 10% is 200 calories. This translates into about one pound (about four servings) of fresh fruit per day — more or less, depending on the caloric density of the fruit. For example, 200 calories can be provided by any of the following: 0.5 pound of bananas (two medium-sized bananas), 0.7 pound of grapes (a big handful), one pound of oranges (three medium-sized oranges), or 1.5 pounds of strawberries (a medium-sized bowl).

However, you do not have to track the calories. Generally, the calorically denser fruits will satiate faster, therefore you will tend to eat less without even trying. Unlike cooked and concentrated foods, fresh fruit gives you a good clear stop signal when you have eaten enough to suit your needs. In other words, you can just eat the amount of fruit that feels right to you, and just leave it at that. Yes, it is that simple to use fruit as a staple food.

Most dietary systems mentioned in this chapter, including the low-carb diets, would allow for about one pound of fruit per day — though some would do so grudgingly. Beyond that, you still have permission to eat all the fresh fruit you want. That permission comes from inside you. Eat fruit conservatively or liberally, in accordance with your constitution and your inner guidance. I am of the opinion that your own instincts and life experiences are your best teachers in this matter.

How to Invite More Fruit and Greens into Your Life

If you have eaten fruit sparingly in the past, and now feel inclined to explore the possibility of using fruit as a staple food, here are some options.

Level 1: Snacks and smoothies (1-3 pounds of fruit per day)
- Prelude to breakfast: 6-12 ounces of freshly squeezed orange juice or grapefruit juice.
- Mid-morning "Coffee Break:" A bowl of strawberries, blueberries, blackberries.
- Mid-afternoon snack: One or two apples, or a bunch of grapes.
- After work or exercise, or before dinner: Fresh pineapple — cut up or blended.
- Anytime snack or light meal: A smoothie made of blended fruit and low starch vegetables. Adjust the proportion of fruits and vegetables to suit your needs.

Level 2: Approaching a high-fruit diet — 3 or more pounds of fruit per day.

If you have played with level 1 for a few months, and feel drawn to explore level 2, you may use any of the following options.

- Continue to use the level 1 options, as you feel inclined.
- Fresh fruit for breakfast. Eat one or more types of fruit, unprocessed or cut up in a bowl. You may also blend the fruit into a delicious smoothie, with vegetables, if you wish.
- Fresh fruit for lunch. Fill up on fruit, or use it as the first course, to be followed by your more typical food.
- Fruit for dinner. Use fruit as the first course, to be followed by your more typical food.

Eating fruit at the beginning of a meal may seem unusual — most individuals have been conditioned to think of fruit as dessert. There is nothing wrong with eating a small amount of fruit for dessert, if you find that you can do so without gastric distress. As you may recall, eating a substantial amount of fruit *after* a heavy meal may cause fruit to stall in the stomach, and ferment.

However, eating fruit *prior* to the heavier foods is an entirely different matter. In fact, if the fruit is acidic or rich in digestive enzymes, it can actually *promote* digestion of the heavier foods that follow. For example, if you eat pineapple or kiwi as an appetizer or the first course of your dinner, the acid and enzymes in the fruit can assist in digesting the fat and protein in the second course.

The key to applying level 1 or level 2 in a healthy manner is simply this: Do it only if you feel inwardly inclined to do so, and proceed slowly.

Note: individuals with blood sugar issues, such as type-2 diabetes, who wish to increase fruit consumption, should monitor their blood sugar, or consult with a health-care practitioner who knowledgeable on the subject.

Chapter 10
Okay, Let's Eat

In the Introduction of this book, I offer two basic guidelines for healthy eating:
- Eat what your instincts tell you to eat.
- Eat an abundance of fruits and vegetables.

These two guidelines go very well together. Fresh fruits and vegetables are the easiest to monitor by our instinctual food radar. When the diet includes enough fresh and minimally processed fruits and vegetables, your instincts are playing in their home field, and can more easily guide you in eating any other foods to complete your nutritional picture. Let those same instincts participate, as we now walk through the process of choosing from the dietary options described in the preceding chapter.

For those who favor the low-carb approach, an easy option is the Weston A. Price Diet, because it allows all the food groups but is very focused on quality. You just have to be mindful about not over-consuming high fat and high protein animal products, or creating deficiencies of the many vitamins, minerals, and phytonutrients found in plant foods. As an alternative, the Paleolithic Diet might fit the bill for those who choose to go easier on the animal fat, while eliminating dairy, and allowing for more fruits and vegetables. Also, be aware that any low-carb diet can be modified to get the majority of calories from plant foods, while still being low-carb.

For those who favor the low-fat approach, the Macrobiotic Diet or Pritikin Diet might fit the bill. Just be careful you do not overdo it on the grains, salt, and soy-based condiments, which are commonly used in these kinds of diets. For the individual who is more motivated, a diet such as Dr. Fuhrman's Eat to Live Diet, with its greater emphasis on fresh fruits and vegetables, might be more appealing.

Also, be aware that you do not have to remain "loyal" any diet. Your responsibility is to your body, which means that your primary loyalty is to the truth of what your body needs. That truth can change with time, because your body changes with time. You might first do well with a low-carb approach, but later feel compelled to switch to the low-fat approach — or vice versa. In that regard, the South Beach Diet offers a good model of how to transition from one to the other.

As a point of caution, when you consider any of the various diets, be aware that even the well-established dietary systems are sometimes modified in response to new findings and challenges that were not anticipated by the founders. For example:

- The Atkins Diet has been modified to include more vegetables and even some fruit.
- The Pritikin Diet has eased up on the consumption of grains, and no longer restricts the consumption of fruit.
- The Paleolithic Diet has evolved into a system that now allows occasional meals that include starchy foods and grains.
- Some vegetarian authors have acknowledged they occasionally eat fish or take supplemental fish-oil.[1]
- Some of the raw food educators have modified their teaching to allow for a modest amount of cooked food.

There is nothing wrong with any of these. It is certainly not a sign of weakness to change your mind in the face of new information. On the contrary, it is a sign of integrity. For the health seeker, the lesson in all this is to simply question authority. The information offered by the presenters of a given diet might be useful, and may have legitimate science to support it, but experience has shown us that the high degree of certainty with which the authors initially present their case is often unjustified.

The signature of good science is candor and caution. The signature of bad science is censorship and the tendency to present theories as facts. This is how we distinguish real science from slick salesmanship wearing a white lab coat.

In other words, a given diet, no matter how convincing it sounds, could have hidden flaws or unseen gaps. It might work beautifully for one individual and be problematical for another. It might initially give you lots of energy and promote rapid weight loss, but lead to problems in the long run.

Any dietary system is useful only to the extent you remember that the ultimate decision maker is you — for the obvious reason that *you* are solely responsible for your health. This important job, in my opinion, should not be delegated to any external authority, because no one knows you better than you.

Time to Choose

If we grew up eating only perfectly natural foods in a perfectly natural environment, food choices could be based entirely on instinct. However, instinctual eating is more challenging when we cook and mix foods. One way to make it easier is to simply choose from a list, rather than having to pull the information out of the "ethers."

Your innate intelligence does not abide by any doctrine. Neither is it contrary to any doctrine. Its usual mode of operation is simple: It guides your educated intelligence in using whatever information is in front of you. In other words, as you encounter choices in the external world, your innate intelligence responds with a silent (or not so silent) "yes" or "no." It may give you the answer right away, or it might do so later, when your rational mind is relatively quiet, such as when you first awaken in the morning.

Below is a chart of the major diets described in the previous chapter. Let your eyes casually scan the list. To keep it simple, do not try to figure out which one "is right" in the absolute sense, but rather ask yourself, "Which one is right for me."

Name	Type	% Carbs	% Fat	%Protein
Atkins	Low Carb	5-20	60-75	20-30
Westin A Price	Low Carb	10-35	45-60	20-30
Paleo	Low Carb	22-40	28-47	20-35
Zone	Low Carb	40	30	30
Blood Type	Mixed	35-65	15-45	15-25
South Beach	Mixed	30-55	20-40	15-25
Macrobiotic	Low Fat	55-65	15-20	10-15
Pritikin or Ornish	Low Fat	80	8-12	8-12
Raw (high fruit)	Low Fat	70-90	5-25	5-10
Raw (low fruit)	Usually low carb	10-45	40-70	7-12

Once you feel that you have a general sense of direction, creating your meal can be fairly simple. The meal options given below include choices that can accommodate all of the major dietary systems discussed in chapter 9, and may be adjusted, as you see fit. In general if your goal is good digestion or weight control, avoid eating large amounts of high carb foods and high fat/protein foods in the same meal.

Breaking the Fast

Morning is a transition time between cleansing and nourishing, and can set the tone for the rest of the day. For this reason, breakfast has been called "the most important meal of the day." However, this does not necessarily mean the meal has to be a heavy one. In fact, for some individuals, breakfast is the most important meal to skip altogether!

The advantage of delaying your first meal of the day is that it offers a greater opportunity for the body to cleanse itself and rebalance. If your body wants an extended "downtime" period, it will give you the signal by simply not registering hunger. Obey that signal by simply abstaining from food, until you are actually hungry.

However, if the inner signal to eat has become a bit weak or hyperactive, here is a rule of thumb: Individuals with any sort of blood sugar issue generally do well with a breakfast that includes a goodly amount amounts protein and fats, or unrefined complex carbohydrates.

As a point of caution, regardless of the condition of your body, skipping breakfast means you have to tap into your reserves of vitamins, minerals, and fuel. This is not a problem if your tanks are full and get refilled daily. However, if the body is already depleted (which is fairly common), skipping breakfast altogether will deplete it even more. This is when the body secretes stress hormones to "get you going." Later in the day, the blood sugar is likely to fluctuate, triggering tiredness, irritability, and mood swings. Therefore, the individual might crave sweets or overeat.

If you feel that you require a hearty breakfast, you are probably right. You can create such a breakfast, using either the low-fat or low-carb approach, as described below. Also, if you have blood sugar issues, I would suggest that you consult with a qualified health professional before making any major dietary changes. With blood sugar issues, in general, minimize or avoid fruit juice and dried fruit, and favor fresh lower-glycemic fruits, such as berries, cherries and apples.

Low-carb Meal Options

Breakfast

1. If you favor a hearty breakfast, start the day with 6-10 ounces of freshly squeezed orange or grapefruit juice, or lemon juice in warm water (include as much as of the pulp as possible). The heavier foods that follow might be 2-3 eggs, prepared according to your taste. In general, any sort of breaking and frying will introduce more oxidation to the fat component of the egg. Soft-boiled eggs are the cleanest and

most nutritionally intact. Next are hard-boiled eggs. With your eggs, you can have breakfast meat or one or two thin slices of whole grain toast with dairy butter or nut butter. Instead of the toast, you can have a small portion of organic grits, millet, or oatmeal. In other words, you can be *very* low-carb, or moderately low-carb.
2. For a lighter breakfast, start with freshly squeezed citrus juice, as above, followed by either dairy or coconut yogurt. Fruit, nuts, and seeds may be added.
3. Start with citrus juice, followed by a bowl of raw organic nuts/seeds and some fresh or dry fruit. It is best to soak the dry fruit, nuts, and seeds for easier digestion. Some seeds may also be sprouted.
4. For an even lighter breakfast, you can have a bowl of fresh organic fruit, either mixed fruit, or better yet, a fruit mono-meal, consisting entirely of one type of fresh fruit.
5. A tall glass of freshly squeezed vegetable juice, including green leafy vegetables.
6. A tall glass of blended vegetables with enough fruit to make it tasty.
7. A quick green drink consisting of water and barley grass powder. If you have a substantial gluten sensitivity, you may use other freeze-dried greens, instead of barley grass.
8. Those who go to work or school can have freshly squeezed orange or vegetable juice in the early morning and an easy-to-mix green drink or fresh fruit as a mid-morning snack. Fresh berries (blueberries, raspberries, strawberries, blackberries, and kiwis) or other in-season fruit would make an ideal mid-morning snack.

Lunch

Some of the lunches described below can easily be prepared in the morning and taken to work. If preparing lunch in the morning does not work for you, the good news is that healthy eating is becoming more popular, and many restaurants offer soups, salads, and sandwiches as healthy "fast foods."
1. Baked fish, chicken, turkey, or beef with assorted steamed or sautéed vegetables, such as broccoli, cauliflower, carrots, string beans, or other veggies as you want. You can also include high quality cultured vegetables (see appendix). If you want to be more moderate with the meat, you can include a small amount of brown rice or a sweet potato.

2. Same as above, but replace the vegetables with a hearty vegetable soup, with an option for a small amount of rice or whole grain bread.
3. A large vegetable salad topped with chicken, fish, cheese or eggs, tofu, tempeh or nuts and seeds. May also include small amounts of brown rice, bread, winter squash, potato, or sweet potato.
4. One or two whole grain pita (pocket) sandwiches filled with any of the following: tofu, tempeh, nut butter, peanut butter, eggs, cheese, or meat. The pocket sandwich can also include raw or cultured veggies on the side or in the pocket. The meal can also include a side dish of chicken soup or beef stew.
5. Here is an option for those who want to seriously eat more fruit and still eat low-carb. Start your lunch with the fruit of your choice. Use the fruit as a light appetizer or the first course, to be followed by any of the options given above. When fruit is used in this manner, it will not be stalled in the stomach and produce gas and bloating. In fact, as previously mentioned, acidic or enzyme-rich fruit, such as oranges, kiwi, pineapple, or papaya will assist in digesting the fat and protein that follow. If you have time, let the fruit "settle" for about 15 minutes before proceeding to the second course.

Dinner
1. Baked or grilled fish, chicken, turkey, or grass-fed beef, with an abundance of steamed, sautéed, or cultured raw vegetables, such as broccoli, carrots, zucchini, beets, and green beans. If you want to be more moderate with the meat, you can include a small amount of brown rice or (real) sourdough bread dipped in melted herb butter or olive oil.
2. Meat and vegetable stew with a salad. You can also reduce the meat a little and replace it with small amount of rice or wholegrain bread.
3. A large salad made with any combination of the following: Shredded romaine lettuce, finely grated carrot, beet, and celery. You can also add larger pieces of softer things, such as sliced tomato, cucumber, zucchini, yellow squash, and green onions. Cultured vegetables can be included. You can sprinkle on any of the following: Chunks of fish, chicken, raw organic goat cheese, hard-boiled egg, avocado, nuts, seeds, tempeh, or olives. The dressing can be as simple as olive oil and lemon juice. Or you can also add a bit of dill, garlic powder, and salt, thickened with ground up flax seeds. Instead of flax seeds, you can use other ground

up nuts or seeds such as hemp seeds, almonds, sunflower seeds, pumpkin seeds, walnuts, or macadamia nuts.
4. Begin with an appetizer or first course of blended or cut-up pineapple (or some other acidic fruit). The rest of the meal can consist of any of the above options.

Low-fat Meal Options

Breakfast
1. If you favor a hearty breakfast, start the day with 6-10 ounces of freshly squeezed orange or grapefruit juice, or lemon juice in warm water, (include as much as of the pulp as possible), followed by whole grain hot cereal, (oatmeal, buckwheat, quinoa) with or without 1-2 eggs.
2. Citrus juice, as above, followed by whole grain cold cereal with organic milk or nut/seed milk.
3. Citrus juice followed by whole grain toast with raw nut butter (tahini, almond/walnut/pumpkin seed/sunflower seed butter).
4. Start with freshly squeezed orange juice, followed by a bowl of raw organic fruit and maybe small amounts of nuts and seeds.
5. A bowl of fresh organic fruit.
6. A tall glass of freshly squeezed vegetable juice, or a quick green drink consisting of water and barley grass powder or other powdered greens.

Lunch
1. A large vegetable salad, with second course of rice and beans, whole grain bread, or potato. As an option, the salad may have a light topping of meat, hard-boiled egg or cheese, nuts and seeds.
2. Rice and black beans with steamed or sautéed broccoli. You can replace the black beans with other legumes, such as lentils or black-eyed peas.
3. One or two whole grain sandwiches made with sliced bread or pita. Fill them with one of the following: tofu, tempeh, natto, nut butter, or peanut butter. The meal can also include raw veggies such as romaine lettuce, tomato, and alfalfa sprouts. For extra flavor and moisture, you can swipe on some butter, mayo, or mustard.
4. One sandwich (regular or pita), plus vegetable soup or small salad.

5. Start with the fruit of your choice. If the fruit tastes really good and you are feeling adventurous, you may eat until you are full. Otherwise, use it as an appetizer or first course, to be followed by a second course consisting of any of the above options. If fruit is used as the appetizer or first course, the ideal plan is to favor acidic or enzyme-rich fruit, such as oranges, kiwi, pineapple, or papaya) because they will assist in digesting the protein and fat in the second course. If you have time, let the fruit settle for 15 minutes before proceeding to the second course.

Dinner

Whole grain pasta and a side dish of beans and steamed or sautéed vegetables. You may also include an assortment of high-quality fermented vegetables. For the pasta, some wheat alternatives include spelt, buckwheat, and rice noodles.

1. Rice and beans with steamed, sautéed, or cultured vegetables, seasoned with tamari. Instead of beans, you can use tofu or tempeh, which you can steam or sauté with the veggies. Or you can simply add the tempeh without steaming to preserve the nutrients that were produced through fermentation. As a variation, you can replace the soy products with a small amount of fish or chicken.
2. A large salad made with any combination of the following: romaine lettuce, grated carrot, beet, and celery. You can also add larger pieces of sliced tomato, cucumber, and zucchini. You can also sprinkle on any of the following toppings: Small chunks of fish, chicken, raw organic goat cheese, hard-boiled egg, avocado, nuts, seeds, tempeh, or olives. The dressing can be as simple as olive oil and lemon juice. Or you can also add a bit of dill, garlic powder, and salt, thickened with ground up flax seeds. Instead of flax seeds, you can use other ground up nuts or seeds such as hemp seeds, almonds, sunflower seeds, pumpkin seeds, walnuts, or macadamia nuts. If you get the dressing right, you can make an entire meal of the salad, using all raw ingredients, if you wish.
3. Quick and Semi-raw: Leftover cooked rice and sprouted lentils, mung beans, or adzuki beans, seasoned with tamari and a dash of organic olive oil. You might be surprised at how tasty it is. You can also include a quick side dish of grated carrots and shredded zucchini topped with miso dressing.
4. See option 5 in the lunch section.

How *Much* Should I Eat?

The old cliché, "All things in moderation," is useful as long as we also apply it to moderation itself. In this case, the need for moderation depends on the food in question, as well as the person. Some individuals seem to be able to instinctively know what and how much to eat, without having to intentionally regulate or restrict portion sizes.

The need for moderation or regulation arises as we alter food from the way it is presented by Nature. When the altered food is also calorically very dense (which is usually the case), we tend to exceed our caloric need before we feel "full," resulting in weight gain. Let's examine each of the food groups in terms of the need to regulate consumption.

Low-starch Vegetables

This category refers to leafy greens, as well as the non-sweet botanical fruits, such as cucumbers, yellow squash, zucchini, tomatoes, and bell peppers. Raw unprocessed low-starch vegetables tend to be low in calories and high in vitamins, minerals, and phytonutrients. Therefore, the need to practice moderation is virtually zero. The real challenge with vegetables is to make sure that you get enough! The same applies to cooked vegetables, provided they have not been batter-dipped, deep-fried, and doctored up with spices and condiments that promote overeating. Cooked vegetables are easier to eat, but generally don't provide the full spectrum of nutrients or the cleansing power as raw vegetables. Blending and juicing are two ways of getting more raw vegetables without having to spend a big chunk of your day grazing.

Starchy vegetables

Starchy vegetables, such as potatoes, sweet potatoes, and winter squash, generally do require some regulation, because they are high in calories and relatively low in micronutrients — the reverse of what we see in low-starch vegetables.

The caloric content becomes effectively higher when the foods are cooked, which is how we usually eat starchy vegetables. Furthermore, since starch is bland, we generally add condiments, such as salt, pepper, MSG, butter, sour cream, or vegetable oil, which can greatly increase the caloric content and toxic residue, while stimulating us to eat more than we would have otherwise. Therefore, we might need to consciously limit the potato portion of the meal, and satisfy the remainder of our appetite with a generous helping of low-starch vegetables, such as a big plate of steamed broccoli and/or a nicely dressed salad.

Fruit

Regarding fresh fruit, the need to practice moderation depends on the individual's ability to effectively regulate blood sugar and metabolize fructose. Under ideal conditions, the individual might be able to eat as much fresh fruit as desired. Dry fruit and fruit juice have sugars in concentrations beyond what we would encounter in Nature; therefore, they should be eaten in small amounts.

What are the ideal conditions that allow for the unrestricted eating of fresh fruit? For practical purposes, there are four main points to consider:

- Physical activity tends to stabilize blood sugar. Therefore, as you increase your level of exercise, you can eat more fruit without maxing out your capacity to process sugars.
- Stimulants induce the adrenal glands to secrete more cortisol, which can contribute to insulin resistance. Caffeine and MSG are the two commonly used substances that stimulate adrenal glands. Therefore, using stimulants on a regular basis is likely to compromise blood sugar regulation.
- In addition to the stimulants in food, anything else that stresses the body, such as emotional unrest, can contribute to insulin resistance and blood sugar issues.
- As dietary fat increases, absorption of blood sugar into the cells tends to slow down.

Grains

Chapter 4 has a detailed description of the potential problems with grains. About 10% of humans are believed to have gluten sensitivity. This, to me, is a signal to the rest of us to limit our consumption of glutenous grains. If you experience any negative reactions at all from eating wheat or any other grain, you might want to just avoid them altogether. However, most individuals can handle the low-gluten and non-gluten grains, such as rice and millet. In addition, amaranth, quinoa, and buckwheat may be used. However, even if you seem to handle grains fairly well, keep the portions moderate, so as leave ample room for those low-starch veggies.

Legumes

Legumes, like grains, are seeds, which means they are calorically dense and contain varying amounts of phytate, which is said to inhibit the absorption of some minerals. However, their overall micronutrient profile is good, and they have been associated with lower rates of cancer and cardiovascular disease. They also provide an alternative source of protein for individuals who want to limit or avoid animal products.

The presence of gas, associated with legume consumption, is one sign that moderation is appropriate. If you handle legumes fairly well, and feel drawn to eat them on a regular basis, simply monitor your reaction and limit your portions so as to silence the gastro-intestinal rumblings. About 1-2 cups of cooked beans provides a substantial amount of calories, protein ,and micronutrients, while leaving room for those low-starch veggies.

Nuts and Seeds

Nuts and seeds tend to be calorically dense and very high in fat. However, moderate amounts in the diet have been associated with reduced incidence of cardiovascular disease and certain cancers. They are a source of omega-3 fats, and some vitamins, minerals, and phytonutrients, as well providing a little added protein for those who want to limit animal products. A proper amount is 1-4 ounces (a small handful) per day, 3-5 days per week, depending on the individual.

Animal Flesh

As with starchy vegetables and grains, meat is high in calories and low in most micronutrients. More specifically, meat is high in fat and protein and relatively low in most vitamins and minerals, and completely lacking in phytonutrients. Since animal flesh packs a lot of calories, we can easily fill up on it to the point that we have little room for anything else. Also, as discussed in chapter 5, the digestive load and toxic residue of animal flesh tends to be higher compared to plant-based foods.

The good news is that we do not have to consume large amounts of animal flesh to get significant amounts of protein and the other nutrients often lacking in plant-based foods, such as DHA and vitamin B_{12}. However, I will refrain from suggesting specific portion sizes, because I am not entirely clear what is driving the great diversity in individual preferences with this food group. In other words, I cannot say for sure where to draw the line between conditioned "cravings' and actual nutritional needs.

Therefore, I will simply remind the reader of the general rule of thumb for any cooked and calorically dense food: Do not just "fill up" on it. Eat the steak or chicken slowly enough to give your brain time to know what's happening. And, of course, leave ample room for those veggies. Other than that, I respectfully place the meat ball entirely in your court.

Eggs and Dairy

As with animal flesh, eggs and dairy are high in calories, which are provided mostly or totally by protein and fat. They are also low in most other nutrients. Therefore, eat them in moderation, while leaving room for the foods that provide the missing nutrients.

If you feel inclined to eat eggs, choose the high quality eggs with the deep orange yolk. If the only eggs you can find are the ones with the runny yellow yolk, I suggest that you consume them sparingly, if at all.

Consuming dairy in a raw and fermented form does seem to make it more user-friendly, especially if it is made from goat's milk, instead of cow's milk. However, if you have any negative reactions to dairy, such as stuffy nose, bloating, or joint pain, you would probably do well to avoid it altogether. Furthermore, since these adverse reactions are so common, as with wheat, I see it as a sign that the rest of us would benefit from limiting consumption of this food.

Food Extracts

Commonly used food extracts are tofu, cheese, butter, olive oil, corn oil, soybean oil, and safflower oil. To this list, we may also add dry fruit (water removed), fruit juice, and vegetable juice (fiber removed).

Food extracts are not whole foods; therefore, they are unnaturally high in some nutrients and deficient in others. Therefore, they can easily create toxicity or deficiency if consumed in large amounts.

The vegetable juice is probably the most use-friendly of the extracted foods. The only real issue with vegetable juice is that it could deprive you of needed fiber — if you rely on it exclusively as your source of vegetables.

If you enjoy tofu, butter, or cheese, and seem to handle them fairly well, use them judiciously, as part of an overall diet that relies mostly on whole foods — which will tend to even out the artificial highs and lows created by food extracts. The good news is that food extracts are so concentrated that you really do not have to consume very much to receive whatever nutritional benefits they have to offer.

What If I'm Still Totally Confused?
Eat just fruits and vegetables until you feel inclined to eat something else.

Part III
THE BIGGER PICTURE

Emotional Eating and Instinctual Eating

How the Author Eats

The Ethics of Eating

Summary and Final Musings

A Journey of a Thousand Miles

A major dietary change is, for most individuals, a rather long process. It is an inner journey into an unknown land. Go on that journey only if and when it calls to you.

When you finally do take the first step, go slowly. This will give your body time to acclimate to the new territory. Beware of the short cut that is actually a detour, or dead end. If you try to move too quickly, you will more than likely end up slowing yourself down. You might injure yourself, or you might get lost.

Be prepared to make course corrections. The maps and instructions, such as this book, might be useful, but they do not replace your own innate sense of direction and personal experience. Regarding your personal needs, remember that your own innate intelligence is always smarter than the teacher's educated intelligence.

Beware of promises of an easy and fast trip to a wonderland of perfect health and delicious food. Such claims are the result of authors trying to answer the public's demand for immediate gratification. Sooner or later, we learn that instant anything is junk.

Companions make the journey easier. However, it is best to go at your own pace. Be mindful of the temptation to speed up or slow down, or the tendency to lose sight of your personal path, in your efforts to cling to your companions.

It is especially tempting to lose sight of your path when you see so many others following another path. The pull of the herd is very strong. However, in the natural world, even herding animals become staunch individualists when it comes to eating. Eat what your body wants to eat. Eat when your body wants to eat. Feasting with family and friends is one of the joys of life, which is hindered only by the odd quirk of thinking we all have to eat the same food in order to belong.

Yes, the path to freedom might feel lonely at times. Along the way, companions come and go. Just say goodbye and say hello. Follow your own path and respect that of others. This is how you can make the journey as pleasant and peaceful as possible, and maximize your enjoyment of the party with all of your fellow travelers on the other side.

The previous chapters address the purely nutritional and logistical parts of one's personal food journey. The remaining four chapters address the less obvious factors — which are ultimately of equal importance.

CHAPTER 11

Emotional Eating & Instinctual Eating

If healthy eating still feels somewhat challenging to you, the issue may very well be the subject of the present chapter. Most of the dietary challenges I have encountered with my patients and myself were clearly related to the presence of emotional needs projected on to food.

Your own emotional nature might be the single most powerful factor that determines the level of success you experience with any diet. Deep inside, you probably already knew this. That is why you might be inwardly nodding your head right now.

There are a number of ways of logically explaining why eating tends to be so emotional. The explanation that is most relevant to food selection has to do with the other major topic of this chapter — instincts.

Understanding Instincts

Instincts are all about survival. Instincts are part of our *innate* intelligence, which means they are, literally, inborn. However, instincts are intimately connected with emotions — and emotions can be programmed. When emotions are programmed in the wrong way, they "scramble" our access to our instincts, so that the latter can no longer serve us.

Since our instincts are connected with emotions, they should be approached with thoughtfulness and care. The key words that describe the process of awakening our instincts are *allow, invite, encourage, nurture, patience, kindness, permission,* and *trust.*

If we can even speak of our instincts as "developing," it is with the understanding that such development is *allowed* to occur organically from within, as with a tree or a field of flowers. As with our emotions, if we try to force our instincts to emerge, or perform on command, they shrink away even further. As pointed out by Henry David Thoreau, "A plant that is not allowed to grow according to its own nature dies; as so a man."

As with our emotions, we cannot "train" our instincts, but rather, we *invite* them to come forth. Just as we cannot make a plant grow faster by pulling on it, we cannot force, but merely *encourage* our instincts, by simply allowing them to be as they are. We *nurture* them by conducting ourselves in a way that gives them *permission* to express. We cannot make them perform on command, but rather "tune" the rational mind to our inner signals by practicing *patience, kindness, and trust*.

We can legitimately speak of challenging and training our rational mind. As with our muscles, the intellect is at its best when it is challenged through the discipline of regular exercise. On the other hand, instincts are more like our internal organs, which function best when allowed to do so according to their own timing and rhythm. Perhaps that is why we often refer to instincts as "gut feelings."

We can apply the above analogy even further. Just as our muscles and internal organs work at their best when they do so in synergistic relation to each other, so do our intellect and instinct. Exercising our muscles regularly and vigorously has been shown to support the health of our internal organs. Likewise, when we allow our internal organs to function according to their own nature, they empower our muscles with vibrant health and energy that galvanizes our physical exercise. The same sort of synergy exists between our intellect and instincts. The right use of intellect allows for the emergence of instincts, which, in turn, bless the intellect with clarity and discernment.

How to Nurture Your Instincts

In essence, we invite the integrative power of our instincts when we quiet the intellect. However, quieting the intellect is not the same as shutting it down. Quieting the intellect means that it is more attentive, and more capable listening to your inner signals.

Quieting our thoughts might be easy to talk about, but the doing of it is usually as easy as trying to make yourself sit still and not think about a pink elephant. Here is the simple answer: The rational mind tends to *spontaneously* quiet down when it recognizes its own limitations, and cultivates the fine art of just being honest about it.

Bringing forth your instincts is not about meditation (although that can help). It's about self-reflection and being honest — especially with oneself. The same honesty that promotes good science also compels the intellect to quiet down. This is how the intellect gradually trains itself to be attentive to the deeper instinctual knowledge that can fill the gaps in the educated knowledge. This is how the intellect and instincts can dance together as Nature intended.

In other words, this is not about the intellect taking a back seat to instincts, or vice versa. It is all about allowing the instinctual nature to emerge from the shadows, and sit next to its natural partner. To the extent we allow this to happen, life is simplified — including the act of eating.

The Eating Instinct

For humans who eat the typical diet of modern civilization, instinctual eating seems unreliable, because foods that taste good don't necessarily promote health. To navigate through this, we simply need to first understand that such behavior does not come from our inborn instincts, but rather from layers of programming that influence or override our instincts.

Such understanding is important, because, if we think that our instincts are the problem, then the solution is to fight or resist our instincts. On the other hand, if we understand that the solution is to *liberate* our instincts, our approach is totally different. Either way, it is not a quick fix. The difference is that if you see it as a need to fight your instincts, you will probably lose. If you see it as a process of liberating your instincts, you will probably win.

The Two Monkey Wrenches

Here are the two main mechanisms that scramble our capacity to receive guidance from our eating instincts.

- **Processed Foods.** Throughout this book, I have pointed out that food consumed by animals in the wild is typically fresh, raw, and eaten one type at a time. In contrast, humans typically cook, mix, and often store food before consuming it. This point is important if we wish to understand why we are often at war with our senses when it comes to food selection. How has the cooking, mixing, and storing of food affected a biological system that has been adapted (for hundreds of millions of years!) to accept food that is fresh, raw, and eaten one type at a time? The answer is that we essentially "trick" our sense of taste. Our nervous system has a harder time "reading" the nutrients, because the molecular language has been changed. Furthermore, through the centuries, we have added an array of condiments, stimulants, and sedatives that trick

our sense of taste even more — refined sugar, caffeine, alcohol, opium, MSG, etc.
- **Processed Humans.** As mentioned earlier, our instinctual food-radar is intimately connected to our ever-present emotions. The emotional connection, in and of itself, is not a problem. In fact, instincts and emotions are supposed to be connected. Our instincts often speak through our emotions, causing us to be drawn to things that are good for us and to be repulsed by things that can harm us. However, when our emotions are traumatized or neglected, we often compensate by using food as a means of experiencing pleasure or numbing the pain. The result is that we eat to fulfill our emotional needs, sacrificing the body's needs.

These two issues tend to reinforce each other. Their connections run deep, and can be traced to a small area deep inside the brain, called the pleasure center. Eating, drinking, falling asleep, physical touch, sex, emotional closeness, creative expression, and spiritual experience all feel good because they are literally "wired" to the pleasure center. When any of these activities no longer stimulates the pleasure center, it no longer feels good, and so we stop doing it.

Ideally, whatever we do to stimulate the pleasure center should promote health and wellbeing. Pleasure, along with pain, is Mother Nature's brilliant invention to get us to do things that promote life. However, when an addiction sets in, we reprogram the pleasure center to be stimulated by activities that do not enhance health.

Exposure to processed foods and emotional stress are two common ways that we unintentionally reprogram our pleasure center. Consequently, the pleasure and comfort of eating no longer necessarily indicate that the body is getting what it needs. Therefore, from a practical standpoint, food selection is a harmonious dance between our innate intelligence (instincts) and educated intelligence (intellect).

Learning to Dance

When it comes to food, the dance between the intellect and instinct is frequently less than harmonious. The two partners seem to bump into each other and step on each other's toes. Ultimately, the educated intelligence is the one that is being the klutz. It makes decisions that essentially disempower the innate intelligence and scramble our food instincts. Furthermore, with our instincts disabled, the intellect becomes even more dysfunctional. Rational thinking, divorced from feelings, becomes rigid, tunnel-visioned, and arrogant. Blinded by its own self-importance and lack of humility, it ultimately becomes self-destructive. Believe it or not, this is relevant to healthy eating.

This book, like other nutrition books, is about providing information for the educated intelligence. However, one of my goals is to provide the information in a way that recognizes the immense importance of the innate intelligence. In this case, healthy eating is not just about gathering information, and has little to do with developing "willpower." It should include an awakening of our eating instincts, which realistically means we must do two things:

- Recognize our conditioned cravings for heavily processed foods.
- Recognize how our nutritional needs have become tangled with our emotional needs.

Each of these two issues, acting alone, is like a monkey wrench that has been thrown into the neurological gears of the brain. However, the simultaneous presence of *both* issues constitutes a double whammy. This is when our willpower crumbles like a house of cards in an earthquake, as we repeatedly revert back to foods we had previously rejected.

How do we remove those two wrenches? The first one (by itself) is relatively easy. We simply walk past the processed foods in the supermarket, and proceed to the produce section. What makes it difficult is the second issue: the tangling of emotional and nutritional needs. Let us, therefore, give some thoughtful consideration to that second monkey wrench — which is often called "emotional eating."

Freedom from Emotional Eating

Firstly, the term "emotional eating" is a bit deceptive because it implies that our emotions have no place at the dinner table. On the contrary, as suggested above, eating is inherently emotional. The act of eating, by design, is supposed to be pleasurable and comforting. The anticipation of eating tasty food is generally experienced as joyful expectancy. The entire emotional atmosphere of the dinner table should not be drab, boring, or mechanical.

Ideally, the emotions that should not be present while eating are those of fear, anger, and sadness, which are, hopefully, properly addressed and resolved before we sit down to eat. The dinner table should not be turned into a battlefield. We should be mindful of its sanctity as a place of peace, relaxation, humor, and joyful sharing.

In the world of the infant, there is an obvious connection between food and emotional comfort. After mother's touch, food is the first form of comfort we experience outside the womb. As we mature, the connection becomes subtler, but still persists.

The intimate bond between emotional comfort and eating must be recognized and respected if we hope to free ourselves from the mysterious and uniquely human habit called "emotional eating"— made even more mysterious by the fact that it has been misnamed. Whatever the name, we simply need to see it for what it is: the habit of relying *too* heavily on food for pleasure and comfort, resulting in the sacrifice of physical health for the sake of emotional gratification.

The present exploration of emotional eating is not intended to separate eating from emotions, but rather to allow the individual to simply recognize where the two have become overly entangled. The rest is mostly an inside job: each individual has to listen deeply and walk gently on his/her personal journey of gradually allowing emotional needs and nutritional needs to loosen their stranglehold on each other, so that both can be fulfilled.

Food and Spirit

To properly understand emotional health, we must understand its relationship to spiritual health. They are not really separate "energies," but rather are part the same continuum of consciousness. Simply put, the two are related in the same way that the child is related to the adult.

When emotional energy is expressed cleanly and honestly, it evolves or "matures" into spiritual awareness. Likewise, spiritual awareness shows up in everyday life as a "rebirth" of emotional innocence, and the capacity to be spontaneous and take joy in the activities of daily living — such as eating!

In other words, *your spiritual life, just like your emotions, has a subtle but powerful influence on how you relate to food.* Most individuals can see how emotional stress can influence how we eat. However, what is less obvious is that a major source of such "stress" is the loss of innocence that occurs when we feel disconnected from our spiritual core.

How do we invite the graceful maturation of our emotions into spiritual awareness? And how do we allow our "spirit" to be born again into our everyday physical reality? That is ultimately a deeply personal and private matter. You are the only person who has the power and authority to choose how you will nurture your soul, just as you are the only one who chooses how to nourish your body.

However, there is a commonality here. When we recognize the limits of our sight, our vision expands. Even if we give no thought to spiritual cultivation, our capacity to "know" anything will expand when we are mindful of what we do *not* know. In other words, we simply remind ourselves that we don't know all there is to know about who we are emotionally and spiritually, just as we do not know everything there is to know about the food we eat. The good scientist would do no less.

With regard to food, the same rational approach that gives us a scientific understanding of nutrition also demands that we frame our body of knowledge against a background of the unknown. The rational mind functions best when it recognizes its own limits. No matter how much we know about human nutrition, we obviously do not know everything! When we lose sight of this, we tend to speak with unjustified certainly, often becoming arrogant and impatient. This is when we fail to see the potential value of nutritional philosophies and opinions other than our own.

By simply recognizing the limit of our sight, we invite an expansion of vision, which quietly shows up as mental clarity and emotional serenity, tempered with a generosity that is neither forced nor strained. We are able to speak from the heart, and respectfully listen to what others have to say. We can sit down and "break bread" with those who see things differently.

In other words, I am not speaking of esoteric philosophies here. This is about the simple willingness to recognize the gaps in our knowledge. This is how we promote sharper discernment. This is how we become more objective, while also inviting the emergence of our natural gentleness and graciousness.

Naturally, the above principle has application well beyond diet and food. However, with regard to this book, I am simply suggesting that, as you consider the purely nutritional information, you also allow your emerging knowledge to be nested within a larger container, which, in practical terms, looks like kindness and respect — towards oneself and others. No matter how important the game may seem, the whole thing becomes meaningless if we forget the dignity and humanity of the players.

In addition to promoting serenity, such an attitude is also likely to enhance your capacity to instinctively know what is nutritionally appropriate for you, even in the face of savvy marketing or social pressures. You will be less likely to trip over your own tangled thoughts and twisted emotions. You will not be so confused by the many differing opinions. Regardless of how "sold" you are on a particular dietary system, you will not become another soldier in the diet wars, but rather maintain the intellectual honesty that allows you to question the concepts you hold as true, while being willing to see the value of other viewpoints.

Such an attitude will help you to remember that your primary responsibility is to your body, which means your primary loyalty is to the truth. More specifically, your primary loyalty is to the truth of what *your* body needs nutritionally. That truth is likely to change over time, simply because the body changes over time. It is entirely possible that the nutritional teaching you reject or ridicule today might have value for you tomorrow.

Emotional Comfort, Spiritual Awareness, and Food Addictions
Yes, the three are connected! As suggested earlier, the heavy reliance on food for emotional comfort frequently shows up as food addictions. The obvious problem with any addiction is that our desires are reprogrammed so they no longer support health and wellbeing. However, there is another, less obvious, consequence of addictive behavior. Any sort of strong addiction tends to delay or arrest emotional maturation. Likewise, the choice to reclaim one's spiritual life is an important step in overcoming any major addiction.

As a point of caution, I wish to emphasize that we must be careful about challenging any firmly ingrained desires, including eating habits. Cursing an addiction does not make it go away, but rather gives it more power. A direct and "willful" assault on our hidden emotional world is generally not successful, and typically does more harm than good.

Even the seemingly harmless process of intellectually examining our food addictions (as we are doing here) must be done with care. To enter the inner domain of one's eating habits is to enter a deep and sensitive area of the mind. It can be a raw and fragile place, which starts to quiver fearfully, putting up a wall of denial, if we approach it with too much urgency or harshness. To attack or reject our conditioned desires in favor of external teachings and dietary ideologies is likely to provoke inner conflict. Such conflict detracts from the potential benefits of a given dietary system.

Kindness is the Key
A change in diet is more likely to succeed if it also includes a change in attitude toward our food choices, an attitude of kindness, supported by patience and respect. I speak here of kindness toward oneself and others. The two are related of course. It is so easy to become impatient with someone else's addictions, when we have not made peace with our own.

As usual, kindness and patience succeed where willfulness and urgency do not. The journey of true dietary transformation is a journey of self-discovery that ultimately goes well beyond food. Such an inner journey is usually not linear and direct, but rather is full of curves and loop-the-loops. It is like a meandering river that follows the contours of the land, sometimes flowing quickly, sometimes flowing slowly, sometimes swirling around in a whirlpool and seemingly going nowhere, as we repeatedly go through our cycles of indulgence and abstinence.

As we float along the river of life on the raft of conscious awareness, not having seen what lies downstream, the only reliable prediction we can make about the journey is that it is not very predictable. Sometimes, the most useful thing the rational mind can do is to remind itself that the river knows where it is going.

The Bigger Picture

Our eating habits may seem totally bad if we use only our educated intelligence to judge the worth of the foods in question. However, when we include our intuition and our capacity to empathize, we tend to see a bigger picture — one that reflects the whole person. That bigger picture might include biochemical, emotional, and spiritual factors unseen by the rational mind. In other words, there might be hidden wisdom behind the seemingly "bad" food choices or "cravings." Therefore, once you have chosen your food, just bless it, give thanks, and enjoy.

As we start to sense that bigger picture, we may eventually see an interesting parallel between nutritional needs and emotional/spiritual needs. Just as the body thrives on whole food, eaten in the manner that Nature presents it, the soul may be said to thrive on the giving and receiving of kindness. Lack of healthy food can contribute to addiction to processed foods, which taste good but harm the body. Likewise, lack of love makes us addicted to drama and conflict, which might "taste good" but do not really nurture, and ultimately undermine our psychological health.

Junk Food for the Soul?

Perhaps you have noticed this about yourself or others: When we deprive ourselves of the opportunity to be loving, creative, and productive, we are likely to drift into fantasy and brooding, rehashing the past, and holding grim expectations for the future. In our daily interactions, we try to build ourselves up by tearing others down. The chronic lack of true friendship causes us to become addicted to the presence of an enemy.

On the larger social level, the addiction can take the form of a perpetual battle against injustice, so we can feel the rush of righteous anger and moral outrage, thus giving us a sense of power and purpose. We shake our heads at the cruel and sadistic acts reported in the news and recorded in history book, but fail to recognize our attraction to such things. On the food front, we become nutrition Nazis, ever on the lookout to expose and criticize dietary imperfections.

Soul Food and Body Food

I share these thoughts because addiction to conflict and addiction to heavily processed foods do not merely parallel each other — they are very much interconnected. To the extent we deprive ourselves of our natural soul food, we will, more than likely, deprive the body of its natural food, as well. Likewise, lack of proper nourishment contributes to mental aberration and emotional turmoil that can translate into conflict and violence.

In other words, if we choose to "clean up our diet," it necessitates the willingness to nourish ourselves on those other levels where we had perhaps been starving ourselves. This is one of the major reasons that so many individuals to go on a treadmill of failed diets and repeating cycles of binging and purging. At some point in our dietary journey, we must tend to the deeper emotional issues and spiritual yearnings that cause us to seek out "comfort foods." When that little detail is handled, the diet we choose can actually work, and the little tricks for promoting instinctual eating, described below, can also work.

How to Awaken the Eating Instinct

- Rediscover mono-eating — one food at a time.
- Be on the lookout for foods that taste good exactly as Mother Nature presents them, with absolutely no mixing, cutting, or processing. In other words, the first contact with the fruit is with your hands, and the second contact is with your teeth.
- Create simple but tasty combinations of unprocessed or minimally processed foods, such as sliced cucumbers topped with dates or sun-dried tomatoes.
- Visit a farmer's market, and rediscover the produce section of the supermarket. Slow down and spend some time there. When you find a fruit or vegetable that really appeals to you, make a meal of it! You can just do this occasionally, whenever you happen to feel like it. If this is right for you, you will probably feel like it more and more often. In

other words, the only discipline you need is the discipline of paying attention to your desires, as you intentionally look for Mother Nature's unprocessed food that is simultaneously appealing to your senses, while blessing your body.

- As you explore the produce section of the store, expand your fruit-seeking vision beyond the usual apples and oranges. Check out the kiwi, cactus pears, fresh figs, blackberries, papaya, persimmons, pomegranates, pineapples, mangos, muscadines, mamey sapotes, dragon fruit, longons, and guavas.
- If you have a garden, rediscover the joy of just picking and eating. If your garden is big enough, you can make an entire meal of it.
- Go to a pick-your-own farm, and allow your nervous system to do what it was made to do — enjoy food right from the tree or vine, surrounded by natural beauty. Most individuals would not think of making a meal entirely of raw and unprocessed tomatoes, lettuce, or okra, but if you pick them yourself straight from the garden, you might change your mind. Food is more satisfying when we pick it and eat it. This is one way you can gently reawaken your capacity to eat instinctively, as well as helping to restore the natural harmony between your nutritional needs and emotional needs. Our instincts for healthy eating work best when we eat straight from the garden — because this is how we were designed to eat!

(Re)Discover Mono-Fruit Eating

For those who are looking for an easy and safe cleansing or weight-loss program, this might be it! Mono-eating is a great way to easily and naturally regulate food intake, because the presence of a single food item at a time gives your nervous system the best possible chance of providing you with a clear stop-signal, when the body has had enough. Even if you feel you have eaten as much as you want of a particular food, but still feel hungry, you can simply stop for a few minutes to give your palate a chance to "reset" itself, and then commence eating another food item.

Mono-eating is what we commonly observe in Nature. Eating one fruit at a time is what we see in anthropoid apes. Likewise, this same practice was probably common among our earliest human and pre-human ancestors.

Even though the author of the Paleolithic Diet does not specifically mention mono-fruit eating, he does say, "eat all the fruit you want." We can imagine how our Paleolithic ancestors may have done just that. Like some modern hunter/gatherers, they might have started their day by filling up on one type of fresh fruit (if available), which would then give them the energy to go out and hunt — without being weighted down and sedated by a heavy fatty meal.

In other words, eating one fruit until full is simply a natural thing to do. We can also do the same with any vegetable if it is tender and juicy enough. The only reason we don't generally do it is because we have been conditioned not to. By using this strategy, you can gently reverse that conditioning and awaken your eating instincts.

Chapter 12
How the Author Eats

I offer this chapter as an example of one individual's nutritional journey — including the all-important emotional and instinctual sides of eating described in the previous chapter. Also, some of the information in this chapter has relevance to the chapter that follows.

If you have read this far into the book, you may have already assumed that my own diet resembles that of other primates in the wild — raw fruits and vegetables, and not much of anything else. Yes, that is pretty much how I eat.

The remainder of this chapter fills in the details of my nutritional journey. I hope you find it useful, but please bear in mind that your own personal needs might be very different from mine, and can change over time.

My Early Childhood

I was born on the Island of Sicily, in a small agricultural village called Raddusa. Most of the open land around the town consisted of rolling hills covered with a tapestry of cultivated farmland — mostly wheat fields, with a *very* light scattering of olive trees, almond trees, and a variety of fruit trees and grape vines. The borders around each property typically consisted of rows of paddle cactus that grew tall and thick wherever allowed to do so.

Yes, the landscape was peaceful and picturesque. Even at an early age, before I knew of any other setting, I found myself appreciating the beauty of the land. Trees were the only things that were in short supply. Lucky for me, close to my house, there was a rare small patch of woodland, where I often played.

In retrospect, I would have to say fruit was my favorite food during my early childhood. My grandfather, as a young man, had created a huge garden of about five acres, containing enormous quantities of vegetables, an abundance of fig trees and grape vines, and a scattering of other fruit trees, such as peaches, oranges, cherries, loquat, mulberries, plums, almonds, and olives. No pesticides or herbicides were used. The only fertilizers were animal manure and ashes from a nearby dump. This garden was the source of virtually all of the fruits and vegetables I ate during the first eight and a half years of my life.

Gardens such as my grandfather's were not very common in that region. Sicily is rather dry, and my hometown did not have an abundance of natural sources of water. My grandfather was successful only because he constructed a holding tank at the highest point in the garden, which was fed by a creek bordering his property. If not for that source of water, and my grandfather's hard work and ingenuity, my diet and my health may have been different in my early years.

The tank was rectangular and made of local rocks and cement. A series of shallow canals dug into the earth conveyed water from the tank to every part of the garden — exclusively through gravity power. At watering time, the attendant removed the stopper from the bottom of the tank, and then walked along with the flowing water, directing its course by pushing dirt around at the points of intersection between any two sections of the garden. I often followed along, totally fascinated by the entire process.

The garden was often buzzing with activity, as people spontaneously gathered to buy produce and socialize. I recall sitting on the terrace, close to the entrance of the garden, with my slightly older cousin, Nicola (named after grandfather), while the attendant took his daily nap in the stone cottage behind us, as my cousin and I enjoyed the cool breeze under the tall shade trees in the quiet of the afternoon.

I spent many a summer afternoon in that garden, eating figs, grapes, and other fruits and vegetables, frequently accompanied by Nicola and, perhaps, some of our other cousins. Between the fruit feasts, we played the usual childhood games. Sometimes, we sat upon the thick wall of the water tank, each of us holding a bamboo pole, as we pretended to be on a boat. We also played Tarzan, among the fig trees and mini-bamboo forests in the garden. Together, we slew many a lion and crocodile and performed other heroic deeds, after which we rewarded ourselves with whatever fruit that was ripe. One memory that stands out was that of Nicola and I climbing one of the huge fig trees, and feasting on amazingly delicious figs, each one almost as big as a tennis ball.

In late summer and autumn, my typical breakfast consisted of cactus pears, usually picked within the hour from a long row of paddle cactus bordering my grandfather's wheat field and garden. The local climate also supported date palms, oranges, apples, pears, and watermelons, all of which I enjoyed, although these other fruits were not as available as figs, grapes, and cactus pears.

I probably ate more fruits and vegetables than most of the other kids in town, because of my grandfather's garden. My oldest brother used to help our grandfather tend the garden and would come home with a bunch of freshly picked fruit and vegetables. Even after my grandfather retired, I remember sitting outside his house in the evenings, with family and friends, illuminated by a doubled-haloed moon and a thick field of stars that included the glowing mist of the Milky Way. There I sat, eating a delicious spiraling cucumber or some other fruit or vegetable that had just been brought up from the garden by the attendant, who often sat with us and told us a story, as he rolled up one of his homemade cigarettes. Telling stories while sharing food was a favored activity during informal social gatherings in those days before television, DVDs, and computer games. I still remember the hearty and satisfying flavor of the cucumbers on those warm summer evenings.

Bread and Fruit

Late summer was especially great because all three of my favorite foods were available. During that time, I think I would have been perfectly happy eating cactus pears for breakfast, grapes for lunch, and figs for dinner. However, my mother obviously would not have that, as I was expected to eat "real food," which consisted largely of bread and pasta. I would say that the bulk of our calories and protein was provided by wheat, supported by various legumes.

The bread was not a problem for me. I enjoyed it and seemed to digest it fairly well. It was probably very nutritious compared to most bread available today. My father grew the wheat, and my mother baked the bread in her igloo oven of stone and mortar.

I am inclined to think that my enjoyment of plain bread and fruit was at least partially due to the local volcano, Mt Etna, the largest in Europe. I found it a bit intimidating with its imposing cone and central crater rimmed with snow, but everyone was basically used to it. It was about 14 miles away, blue and hazy on the horizon — close enough to bless our soil with periodic dusting of mineral-rich ash, but far enough to give us a false sense of security.

The major nutritional drawback to the bread was its lack of bran. By the time I was old enough to remember, the local mill had already become sophisticated enough to remove the bran, which we then fed to our chickens and pigs.

In those days, only the poorest families ate bread with bran. We did not know about the vital nutrients found in bran. We were simple peasants, far removed from the urban mainstream of Western civilization, at a time when

TV and telephones were rare, and the Internet was still some 40 years into the future.

Anyway, I was too young to care about the virtues of bran. The homemade bread we ate was yummy, and that's all that mattered to me. I especially liked it on bread-baking day, when the loaves were still warm from the oven. On those days, we often sliced the bread while it was still steaming hot, and dressed it with olive oil and a few spices. I personally preferred just olive oil, and not much of it. In addition, on bread-baking day, my mother sometimes made a traditional flat-bread called a "fu-atza," which was probably the ancestor of pizza — topped with olive oil, herbs, and spices, and often included a sprinkling of Parmesan or Romano cheese. Pasta, however, was another story.

My Battle with Pasta

For about the first fifteen years of my life, I didn't like pasta in any form. The main problem was the texture, which was flat-out revolting to me. Furthermore, unlike our homemade bread, which was delicious to me all by itself, pasta had no flavor of its own and was usually loaded down with garlic, onions, and other heavy spices, which did not appeal to my simple fruit-and-bread palate.

I had to eat pasta every day, as the first course of our main meal, which typically occurred at around 1:00 PM or 1:30 PM. After that heavy meal, we traditionally took a nap — although I usually preferred to go out and play. For these two reasons (mandatory pasta, followed by a nap), the main meal of the day was not my favorite.

In contrast, the evening meal was more enjoyable to me. It was more modest and informal, consisting of leftovers from the earlier main meal — cooked vegetables and pasta (which I thankfully was not required to eat), as well as the usual bread, olives, cheese, homemade dry sausages (which I didn't like), and whatever fruit that was in season — which I devoured. Like most families, we did not have a refrigerator, so food was typically eaten on the same day it was picked or cooked.

Since I was required to eat pasta seven days a week, I got into the habit of swallowing it whole without chewing, so as to avoid the revolting texture, and minimize my perception of the other gustatory abominations. Swallowing the pasta whole probably did not do anything good to my young digestive system.

Most cooked vegetables were palatable to me, as long as they were not loaded down with garlic, onions, and other strong spices. My favorite part of the main meal was dessert — fresh fruit in the warmer months and dry fruits or roasted chestnuts in the cooler months.

Sometimes we ate meat, such as one of our chickens, for Sunday dinner. However, the more typical animal products consisted of fresh eggs or milk from our animals, and several kinds of locally made cheeses. I did not care for the strong aged cheeses that were commonly used, except maybe when it was sprinkled in small amounts on our homemade proto-pizzas. I did enjoy freshly made (unspiced) ricotta cheese. Homemade ricotta, warm, steaming, still floating in its own whey, and eaten with bread, was one of my winter favorites.

Olives were also a common feature of the local diet. As in the rest of Sicily and other countries that rim the Mediterranean, bread and olives were often combined into a meal or snack — a tradition that goes back thousands of years. One of my uncles ate a diet consisting mostly of homemade bread, home grown olives and, when available, home-grown tomatoes. As far as I know, he suffered no ill effects, and lived to be 90. However, I personally did not care too much for the combination of bread and olives, because the latter were generally cured with a lot of salt, vinegar, and loaded with garlic and other strong spices.

My attitude toward olives pretty much describes my attitude toward any heavily doctored foods. I ate them only when I was coaxed or intimidated to do so. In fact, I can summarize those early years in Sicily, by saying that I thrived on homemade bread and freshly-picked, tree-ripened fruit, along with simply prepared vegetables, while doing my best to avoid most of the other heavily spiced concoctions.

Coming to America

From the day I stepped off the ship, the Italian bread we got from the local bakeries was quite acceptable to me. However, the packaged white bread (advertised for its alleged ability to "build strong bodies 12 ways") was initially more disgusting to me than pasta. In addition to the unappealing texture, the smell was downright revolting to me.

My earliest memories of grade school in the United States include the overpowering smell of white bread and cold cuts in the cafeteria at lunchtime. I found it borderline nauseating. I was grateful that Public School 48 was close enough to allow me to run home for lunch.

Eventually, I did adapt to the new foods, including white bread. At first, I toasted it to dark-brown crispiness, and slathered on peanut butter or jelly (I generally did not like to mix them). Gradually, I was able to eat white bread with less toasting and camouflage. By the time I entered junior high school, which was too far for me to run home for lunch, I actually enjoyed bologna and American cheese on white bread — no toasting, no problem!

By the time I got to high school, I was thoroughly "Americanized," and started eating school lunch on a regular basis. By then, I had long gotten over the intensely disorienting culture shock of moving from a small agricultural village in Sicily to Planet New York City.

Fruit retreated into the background, because it was a far cry from the freshly picked delicious morsels grown on rich volcanic soil, back in the old country. Furthermore, my taste buds were gradually becoming jaded by the once overpowering and disagreeable flavors of processed foods. To satisfy my sweet tooth, oranges were replaced by orange soda, figs were replaced by Twinkies, grapes were replaced by grape-flavored popsicles, and freshly picked cactus pears became a distant memory.

I do not exactly recall when I actually started to be able to chew pasta without being totally grossed out, but somewhere during my latter teen years, my taste buds "matured" enough to be able to appreciate a nice plate of spaghetti or pasta fazul (pasta with beans) — provided the garlic was kept to a moderate level, and the onions were undetectable to my eyes and taste buds. Paradoxically, by then, I did not have to eat pasta every day, because I was often not home for dinner, due to college and my expanding social life. I remember arriving home in the evenings after a late class, and enjoying a plate of leftover spaghetti warmed up in a frying pan, as I watched Monty Python's Flying Circus.

My Chronic Health Issues

Yes, I did get sick a lot in the New World, starting from the early days after stepping off the boat, all the way through my college years. I'm inclined to think that my condition was due to a constitutional weakness, combined with the massive amount of wheat in my diet. Even as a child in Sicily, I periodically found myself in bed with a fever.

As far back as I can remember, my digestive system and immune system were both on the delicate side. The two are very much related, as I later learned. The same enzymatic activity that breaks down food also breaks down pathogens. Furthermore, a big chunk of our immunity comes from the beneficial bacteria and white blood cells in the gut.

It took me many years to discover that the secret to a strong immune system is to reduce the burden on the digestive system. For me, that translated into drastically reducing and eventually eliminating wheat and animal products.

Granted, my Southern Mediterranean heritage allowed me to adequately digest wheat. However, adequate digestion does not necessarily mean that it is well received by the rest of the body.

I suspect that the abundance of fresh fruits and vegetables during the long growing season in Sicily brought a measure of grace to my condition. In retrospect, the diet and lifestyle of rural Sicily during my early childhood were similar to that of the folks on the neighboring island of Sardinia, who have been reputed to enjoy excellent health and longevity, as described by Dan Buettner in his book, *The Blue Zone*.[1] In fact, as I recall, the proportion of people in my home town enjoying good health into their 90s was rather high.

I am reminded here of my oldest brother, who once attended a social gathering of senior citizens in our hometown. During the gathering, one gentleman, proposed a toast: "May we all live to be a 100!" This elicited a protest from one of the older gentlemen in the group. "Wait a minute," he said, "I'm 95!"

When my family immigrated to the USA, we had moved from a small town where the climate was warm, the air and water were clean, and the food was fresh and locally grown, to a big city, where I ate a goodly amount of processed foods, deficient in vitamins, minerals, and phytonutrients. As I grew older, I ate more meals at fast food restaurants. While attending college, I basically lived on burgers, French fries, soft drinks, and milk shakes, like most of my fellow students.

Occasional injections of penicillin to help me fight off the nastier fevers and respiratory infections were part of my life. However, though my health problems often claimed my attention and that of my mother, the connection with food was never made. Our family physician of many years was a kind and competent doctor, but I do not recall him ever correlating my frequent illnesses with diet.

Change in Diet

By the time I was around 24 years of age, the grace of youth started to decline, and I began experiencing bleeding hemorrhoids, part of which could be attributed to years of constipation and straining. At that point, I still knew nothing of nutrition, and the correlation between food and diseases. However, by a happy coincidence, my first teaching job was at a massage school, where I started my long journey of discovery into the hidden causes of my chronic health issues.

Since I was living on my own by then, I had gotten into the habit of eating convenient fried foods, such as fish and chips, fried potato thingies, and chicken nuggets. I eventually noticed that my consumption of these greasy foods coincided with bleeding of my hemorrhoids. I could not understand why fried foods would have such an effect. The medical doctor I finally consulted did not have a clue.

Fortunately, massage school is a gathering place for individuals interested in so-called alternative healing. During that time, I attended a seminar by a chiropractor who introduced me to the idea that fried greasy foods essentially "clog" the liver, and impede the flow of blood through it. This, he said, can lead to bleeding hemorrhoids.

Since I was teaching anatomy and physiology, the chiropractor's explanation made perfect sense to me: The veins from the stomach and intestines take the blood directly to the liver. Therefore, if the liver is clogged with fried greasy food, this could theoretically increase the blood pressure in those veins, in which case the tiny veins in the anus could swell up and eventually break.

The Journey Begins

My liver revelation was my introduction to nutrition. Since then, I have become progressively more interested in the correlation between food and health. Granted, during most of those years of nutritional exploration, I was not above partaking in various culinary delicacies, but as my studies became more focused, my diet evolved accordingly.

By the time I entered chiropractic school, I also began exploring fasting and other methods for encouraging the cleansing and healing of the body. Apparently, I did experience tangible benefits — besides the improved digestion and eventual elimination of hemorrhoids. When I first entered chiropractic school, X-ray films of my spinal column revealed a small calcium deposit just in front of the neck vertebrae. About twelve years later, a subsequent film showed the calcium deposit was gone. This is significant because such growths generally do not dissolve, but rather tend to grow in size.

"Stimulants Weaken You"

In European culture, during my early childhood, there was no strong injunction against kids drinking coffee, beer, or wine. In fact, I remember being encouraged to try all of these at the dinner table. However, as a child, I disliked all three. In retrospect, I did not care for anything that was strongly stimulating or sedating. Such foods were often bitter or pungent, which did not appeal to me. Eventually, as I grew older, I did develop a tolerance for such items, and even learned to appreciate their role as vehicles of social interaction — as well as the nice little "buzz" they can provide Like other adults, I also developed a taste for salt and other spices, even garlic and hot pepper, in moderate amounts.

It was during the early years of nutritional exploration that I received my first hint that I would do well to eat as simply as possible. While in the middle of a three-day fast, I was feeling unusually calm and clearheaded, and a thought flashed through my mind — almost like a voice in my head: "Stimulants weaken you."

I understood, "stimulants" to mean anything that stimulates my nervous system, even if it simply stimulates my appetite — salt, pepper, soy sauce, MSG, garlic, etc. I understood that I should be moderate with the use of any condiment that strongly influences the natural flavor of food. The implication was to find peace, joy, and pleasure in ways that do not over-stimulate or otherwise stress the body.

I was being inwardly guided to a diet and lifestyle advocated by Natural Hygiene (described in chapter 9). I was being guided to favor foods that do not require a lot of strong spices to make them appetizing. Unknown to me at the time, I was being guided toward a simple diet consisting mostly, or totally, of raw and minimally processed food.

My Introduction to Raw Eating

My first modest exploration of raw eating came shortly after I graduated from chiropractic school. I decided to eat just raw food for 40 days. This was well before the current "raw food movement" took hold, with its many books and seminars. Having very few resources to draw upon, my strategy was to start by eating fruits, vegetables, and a few nuts, seeds, and avocados. I focused mainly on juicy fruits and vegetables, since I had already learned these are the most cleansing and non-toxic of the food groups. I then phased out the fatty foods, and, for a few weeks, I ate only juicy fruits and vegetables, and then just fruit. Finally, I ate just watermelon for three days.

Without realizing it, I was playing with what would eventually become my everyday diet. However, following my 40-day raw adventure, for another eighteen years or so, my diet remained predominately cooked, punctuated with an occasional raw cleanse in the summer months.

When I finally decided to take the plunge, by going raw in earnest, I started by attending a ten-day raw food seminar. This particular version of the raw diet featured a goodly amount of sprouts, wheat grass juice, lots of salads, and very little fruit. That is what I ate initially, which allowed for a very nice cleansing of the body, while still providing me with a wealth of vitamins, minerals, and phytonutrients. However, I had to eventually increase my caloric intake so as to be able to maintain my weight. I did this by increasing my consumption of fatty foods — nuts, seeds, avocados, coconuts, and extracted oils. These foods were often in the form of tasty combinations that served as the raw analogues of lasagna, pizza, meat loaf, apple pie, etc.

"Nut Butter Yucky!"

On the high-fat raw diet, I did not experience the improvement in health that had been lead to expect by its teachers. Finally, I received some strong inner signals that seemed to be urging me to modify my eating. One such signal was the onset of arrhythmia (irregular heart beat), which I corrected by increasing my mineral intake — including the reintroduction of some cooked vegetables, grains, and beans.

When I tried to go totally raw again, using the high-fat approach, I received another signal that compelled me to reconsider my choice: Early one morning, while still in a deeply relaxed state wherein the mind is likely to go into a reverie of dreamy images and voices, I saw a bowl of what I took to be nut butter. That, in and of itself, would not have meant anything to me. I would have simply assumed I was seeing nut butter because that was what I had been eating in substantial amounts. However, I also heard a voice — a young child's voice, which clearly and emphatically exclaimed, "NUT BUTTER YUCKY!"

I immediately surmised that I was being strongly advised (in a cutesy sort of way) to drastically reduce my fat intake, especially nuts and seeds. At first, I inwardly "argued" with the messenger. However, as much as I enjoyed nut butter, coconuts, and avocados, I had to admit the message made physiological sense. Even though my problems with bleeding hemorrhoids were well behind me (so to speak), I understood that my grace period would not last much longer, if I continued with my high-fat ways. Yes, these fats were kinder to my liver than the fried fish sticks I used to eat, but I was also consuming the raw fats in larger amounts than I ever had. They were easily providing me with 60% of my daily calories, sometimes more.

Anyway, I grudgingly reduced the nut butters and avocados to much lower levels. However, I was also in a quandary. The playful message from my subconscious mind showed me what *not* to eat on a 100% raw diet, but did not indicate what I *could* eat. So, I went back to cooked food, again.

In retrospect, I suspect I was already closed off from the answer, simply because I had been indoctrinated against it. Therefore, I had to be "ambushed" in a way that circumvented my programming. The ambush came in the form of a book that literally fell on my lap. While I was sitting quietly at home, a friend walked in and gave me a copy of *The 80/10/10 Diet*, by Dr. Douglas Graham. That was when I finally considered a new solution to my raw dilemma — fruit.

When I first looked at the cover of book, I think I experienced a muffled excitement of sorts, like the unrestrained cheering of 70,000 people in a distant stadium. The feeling part of my brain seemed to be saying "Yes!"

However, my intellect needed to be convinced, so I methodically read the book, and then read it again. The explanations as to why it is okay to eat larger amounts of fruit made sense to me, but before I drew any conclusions, I decided to put it to the test. Ever since then, my meals have become simpler and fruitier.

How I Eat Now

For the past eight years, my diet has consisted predominantly of raw fruits and vegetables. I also include small amounts of nuts, seeds, avocados, and coconuts. Occasionally, I use a little cinnamon or ginger, and drink herbal teas. I also periodically take small amounts of vitamin B_{12}. During the colder months, I sometimes take vitamin D. On occasion, I have taken small amounts of algae oil — if I feel the need for additional omega-3 oils. However, whatever benefits I receive from these products seem to be rapidly lost if I use them more than sparingly.

According to the lab tests, my blood sugar, triglycerides, cholesterol, and other markers have been consistently well within normal limits. None of the warnings I have read about regarding the dangers of a high fruit diet have proven to be true for me.

With this diet, overeating is actually difficult for me. If the foods I eat on any given day consist *entirely* of raw and unprocessed fruits and vegetables, the only way I can over-consume calories is to actually force myself to do so. No matter how delicious the fruit, no matter how fresh and tender the vegetables, I eventually reach a point where eating is no longer pleasurable.

Finding Your Truth is Like Returning Home

In retrospect, the evolution of my diet over the course of my life has been, in one sense, a spiraling journey — an intentional return to food choices that resemble the instinctual likes and dislikes of my early childhood. Fruits now provide the bulk of my daily calories, even during those times that I have eaten some cooked foods.

The large amount of fresh fruits and vegetables seems to be gradually transforming my sense of taste to that of my early childhood. For example, my craving for salt has steadily decreased. The use of spices, condiments, and stimulants, which I found most objectionable as a child, but learned to appreciate as a young adult, have gradually decreased — without much effort on my part.

My idea of a perfect meal is now to find a fruit tree in a beautiful and peaceful setting and eat until full, or maybe follow the fruit with a second course of freshly picked raw vegetables — as I used to do in my grandfather's garden in Sicily.

The inclusion of cooked foods is currently still an option for me, although their appearance on my plate has steadily declined. I have eaten them mostly in the winter months. The inclusion of animal products during the past 20 years or so has been infrequent, and has gradually reduced to zero, during my raw years.

However, I will not categorically say I will never go back to animal products or cooked foods. I am willing to include these foods if I become convinced that my health requires them. Even though I have been eating this way for eight years, I still consider my current diet to be an experiment. I also wish to emphasize that my decision to exclude animal products was not based on the persuasive arguments and evidence presented by vegan authors, but rather my own inner signals that have consistently nudged in that direction, as I explain below.

Nurturing My Eating Instinct

Throughout this book, I have advocated the reawakening of instinctual eating, as a vital part of making healthy food choices. I have also suggested that the inclusion of raw and unprocessed fruits and vegetables, especially eaten one at a time, will more than likely promote easier access to our eating instincts.

Have I experienced any noticeable changes in my capacity to receive such inner signals? I would have to say yes. On the most mundane level, I no longer have to consciously "regulate" how much food I consume or how many calories I ingest. I simply eat until full, and seem to maintain my weight, muscle mass, and energy level.

I have also found that if I require any foods besides raw fruits and vegetables, my body lets me know. For example, if I eat just fruits for a few days, I will eventually want some vegetables or vegetable juice. Neither do I have to sacrifice pleasure for the sake of "good nutrition." I eat the specific fruits and vegetables that are most appetizing to me. The only time I have to consciously control the amount of food I eat is when I include nuts, seeds, avocados, coconuts, or cooked food.

In other words, for the most part, my eating instinct shows up in a manner that closely resembles that of any animal in the wild. However, I have occasionally experienced this greater access to my food instincts in more "exotic" ways. As with other humans, I have dreams, hunches, and "gut feelings." When I become quiet and relaxed enough, I sometimes receive signals in the form of an image or a quiet voice in my head, regarding food choice. Here are some examples:

Fruitful Visions
- On two occasions in the early years of my raw food journey, while dreaming, I saw images of small amounts of tofu. I got some tofu (in real life), which I ate and enjoyed, and then happily returned to raw.
- On a few occasions, I have seen small bits of cooked meat or fish, which I eventually decided to eat in real life. As with the tofu, I was happy to give thanks for the novel experience, and then return to raw fruits and vegetables.
- On a number of occasions, I have received images of bananas, even during the first 6 years or so of my raw journey, when bananas did not appeal to me that much. These banana images have often coincided with periods of increased stress. I find this interesting, because bananas have a reputation for promoting relaxation and mood elevation. Over the past year, banana visions have been more frequent. Not surprisingly, during this time bananas has become tastier to me, than they have in the past.
- During the winter months, I have periodically received images of oranges. I do enjoy oranges, but the images have often included a "suggestion" to go easy on this fruit. Sure enough, I have noticed that when I eat a lot of oranges, I sometimes get over-energized or sedated, which are common reactions to low-grade allergens.

Animal Products
During one winter, I found myself eating cooked foods 3 or 4 days of the week. I had also included animal products on a couple of occasions, and was

contemplating having some more. I was not particularly craving animal products, but the idea of eating them was sort of appealing, and I also thought they might be "good for me." I deliberately asked my innate intelligence if I should eat animal products. A few days later, upon awakening, while my mind was still deeply relaxed, and my eyes closed, I received my answer, which came in the form of a single word. That word was, "Vegan."

The following winter, I went through a similar dance. I was eating cooked foods 3 or 4 days a week, and was contemplating eating some cheese or eggs. Once again, I asked for guidance. And once again, the answer arrived in the quiet of the early morning, while still in bed, with my eyes closed. This time the guidance came in the form of two words: "Strict vegan."

Homocysteine

"Homocysteine" is a word that was once whispered in my ear in the quiet of early morning. In retrospect, this one-word message served as a sobering counterpoint to my other signals to follow a raw vegan diet. As you may recall, homocysteine irritates the inner lining of blood vessels, and is proving to be a much more accurate predictor of cardiovascular disease than high cholesterol levels.

High blood levels of homocysteine can be caused by deficiencies in folate, B_{12}, as well as low levels of two amino acids — cysteine, and methionine. Folate is not a problem for me, because I get an abundance of it in the foods I eat. However, the other three can be lacking in my diet. Coincidentally, a subsequent blood test showed that my homocysteine level was less than ideal, though it was still within normal limits. Likewise, my B_{12} level was okay, but still not ideal.

In other words, both my inner signal and blood test pointed in the same direction. Together, they served as a gentle reminder to take action before a potential problem becomes a real problem. My solution: I occasionally supplement with B_{12}, while also making room for raw vegan foods that feature modestly higher levels of methionine and cysteine, such as most nuts and seeds, especially sesame seeds, and some vegetables, such as broccoli, kale, spinach, and zucchini.

Oatmeal Brain

During my most recent winter, I decided to try raw oatmeal, which I prepared by soaking and sprouting whole oats, and then blending them in hot (not to hot) water. To my delight, it tasted just like cooked oat meal. I enjoyed it so much that I contemplated doing the same thing with other grains.

However, the morning following one of those meals, my energy was sort of low, and my mind was sort of foggy and restless. For a while, I wondered if I had reacted to the oatmeal, but eventually forgot about it, as I plodded through my early morning activity. Later that morning, during my meditation, I dozed a little — because I was still tired. In the midst of reverie, I saw an image of my brain. Then, to my surprise, I saw oatmeal being poured on my brain. The message was unmistakable: "This is your brain. This is your brain on oatmeal."

I also understood that the message was not just about oatmeal — which is actually one of the healthier grains we can eat, having a number of beneficial properties. However, I had also previously received other signals, warning me that substantial amounts grain-products tend to "clog" my body and mess with my mind. Since oats is one of the "healthier" grains I can eat, my oatmeal vision underscored the previous signals to go easy *all* grains, or avoid them altogether.

A Message from the Doctor

During another winter, I received a rather unusual message that really got my attention. As in previous winters, I was eating cooked foods 3 or 4 days a week. This time, however, I was also indulging in many of my old comfort foods: cheese pizza, Mexican food, and lots of bread, and other foods that were doctored up with stimulants and spices. Not surprisingly, the voice of wisdom intervened in a more definitive way. It happened while I was dozing. The voice clearly said: "Eat fruits or vegetables."

The message was simple and to the point, and I probably would have forgotten it, if not for the fact that it was delivered in a way that was rich in meaning, wit, and humor. It was like an auditory hologram, which lasted just one second or so, but compelled my rational mind to think about it for days, before I fully grasped its implications. You see, the message was not merely a generic voice in my head, or a clear and lucid thought, but rather came in the voice of a specific real-life person whom I recognized.

It was the voice of an individual whom I will call Dr. R. At the time, the real Dr. R was a United States congressman for the state of Texas. Since I had been following his work, I had developed certain impressions about him — all of which came together to give several levels of meaning to the simple suggestion to eat fruits and vegetables. For example:

- Dr. R had a reputation for being a highly principled and honest politician, who told you the simple truth. In other words, a "straight shooter from Texas" was telling me the truth regarding how I should eat.

- Dr. R was also a real-life medical doctor. Since I would only see a medical doctor if I was faced with a serious health problem, I was essentially being told that I needed to return to my fruit and vegetable diet, or face serious medical consequences.
- Dr. R was a staunch conservative, and was often critical of political liberals. I took this to mean that I should eat simply and conservatively. By implication, I was being told to avoid excesses, and not be too "liberal" and complicated with my meals.
- Around the time that I received my fruits and vegetables message, the real Dr. R was speaking out against the use of a proposed government "stimulus" to boost the economy. He warned that such quick fixes would eventually weaken the economy even more. Why is that significant to *me*? In the past, I had received repeated signals to avoid using stimulants. The voice of Dr. R was reminding me of what I already knew, but had forgotten: "Stimulants weaken you!"
- Dr. R's foreign policy was consistently one of peace and non-intervention. This metaphorically describes the health and wellness strategy that seems most appropriate for me. Over the years, what has worked best for me is to cultivate inner peace, eat simply, and to minimize "intervention" with herbs and supplements to address a given health challenge. Instead, I have been guided to allow the body to gradually and naturally reset itself.

As I contemplated the many facets of that seemingly simple message to "Eat fruits and vegetables," I marveled at the genius and elegance of the inner guide that resides in every one of us. I was reminded that health, happiness, and peace cannot be acquired entirely through external information. With all of its worldly knowledge, the educated intelligence must be able to quiet itself and receive the guidance and blessings of the innate intelligence.

Fitness and Food

As of the time of this writing, I have been on a fitness program for almost a year and a half. Basically, I walk/run 10-30 miles per week. I also generally do some yoga stretches and other exercises in the early morning, prior to my road work.

In addition to endeavoring to improve my overall health, I wanted to see if my higher level of fitness would influence my dietary journey. Prior to starting my fitness training, my occasional return to cooked foods in the winter months seems to have been at least partially (or perhaps totally) emotionally based. What does physical fitness have to do with this? Like many other individuals, I have noticed a correlation between physical exercise and improvement in my mood. Therefore, I figured that by becoming more active, I might possibly experience a higher level of emotional poise, and therefore no longer be seriously tempted by my old cooked comfort foods.

Furthermore, I reasoned that if there *is* a genuine nutritional need associated with my periodic craving for cooked foods, it might be related to my body not yet being able to absorb the necessary nutrients on my low-fat, raw vegan diet. If that is the case, the increase in physical fitness might possibly provide an answer, because regular exercise is known to significantly improve digestion and absorption. The results of my physical training program have been as follows:

- In the first six weeks or so, I went from running a maximum of about one mile (with much huffing and huffing), to running my first race (nine miles) with relative ease and grace. Several months later, I ran my first half marathon. Thus far, I have been too chicken to sign up for a full marathon.
- As expected, I have been feeling physically stronger and more energetic, as well as experiencing a subtle but noticeable improvement in mental clarity and emotional poise. Essentially, the physical training seems to have enhanced the benefits I have already experienced from my simple fruit and vegetable diet.
- On the food side, I have felt significantly more settled on my raw vegan eating plan, and all foods seem to taste better to me. Also, I remained on a totally raw diet this past winter, unlike my previous seven years that I have been on this eating plan.

The Results of My Eating Raw

Here is a summary of the changes I have noted during my years of raw eating.

- My energy is steady. In general, I no longer feel the previously common mid-afternoon lows. I now feel more energetic than I did 20 years ago. I tend to maintain good energy even when I teach a four-hour night class that ends at 10:30 PM, whereas, prior to that, I often turned into a slug at around 9 PM.
- My chronically painful left wrist has greatly improved and is mostly undetectable.

- The occasional pain at the base of the neck from an old injury has virtually disappeared.
- Immune system seems to be much stronger. Prior to starting my raw journey, respiratory issues were a common occurrence, including lower respiratory infections that lasted 2 or 3 weeks. Since then, I have had a moderate respiratory infection on three occasions, two of which coincided with a return to cooked and fattier food.
- My digestion seems to be stronger, and bowel movements more regular.
- Rectal prolapse seems reduced.
- The lipoma (fatty cyst) on my right shoulder gets noticeably softer and somewhat smaller when I stay on a raw, low-fat eating plan, and becomes larger and firmer when I return to cooked or high-fat foods.
- Over the past eight years, my use of herbs and supplements has steadily decreased. My tendency has been to use more herbs and supplements when I return to cooked food or increase my consumption of raw fatty foods.
- The vitiligo (patches of depigmentation on the skin) has started filling in some places.
- Elimination of athlete's foot, jock itch, and toenail fungus.
- Blood sugar, cholesterol, and triglycerides levels have been excellent.
- The only dental work I have received has been for pre-existing issues.
- I no longer experience sensitivity of my teeth, unless I eat enormous amounts of acidic fruit, and even then, it is relatively minor, compared to when I ate predominantly cooked food.

Chapter 13
The Ethics of Eating

Regarding the purely nutritional side of eating, the obvious goal is to promote personal health. In contrast, the ethical considerations are a matter of conscience, having to do with our relationship with the life around us. More specifically, the ethical side of eating compels us to modify our food choices in accordance to environmental, humane, or spiritual considerations.

In general, the underlying simplicity is that the foods that best support personal health are the same foods that can be most easily grown in an ethical and sustainable manner.[1] Anyway, that is how it is supposed to work. However, under our current system, the ethical concerns often prove to be so cumbersome that many individuals resort to avoiding any potential conflict by simply not looking at the ethics of eating. This is not anything to feel guilty about. There are just so many things we can have on our plate at any one time. You know best how to prioritize your life. Just as you have the natural authority to choose how you will nourish your body, you are also the only one who decides if and when you need to consider any of the ethical concerns about food. For those who do feel compelled to give this subject some attention, I offer this chapter.

Which Is It for You?

One way to minimize the misunderstandings, confusion, and conflict that often surround this subject, is for the individual to be clear about his/her personal priorities regarding food selection. For example, if your main priority is physical health, you need not feel guilty about "neglecting" the ethical considerations. Likewise, if you are primarily motivated by the ethical considerations, you would not make the mistake of trying to defend those ethical choices through nutritional arguments, because your choice is a matter of conscience, and does not need (and might actually be weakened) by such defense. If you do encounter nutritional challenges, you would not deny or trivialize them, but rather address them honestly, and then do your best to resolve them in a way that honors your spiritual, humane, or environmental concerns.

Furthermore, when you *do* honestly attend to whichever side that is calling to you most strongly, you will more than likely also be guided to eventually adjust your food choices so as to give proper recognition to the other side. In this manner, your health needs and ethical concerns dance harmoniously and synergistically in your personal life.

Environmental Considerations

The use of dirty methods of food production eventually cycles back to the consumer, who must live on foods that are progressively more toxic and less nutritious. Yet, authorities tell us that the toxic chemicals routinely used in food production are necessary. Is that really true? The answer depends on how you look at it.

It's All in the Soil

Growing clean and nutritious food is not unlike the process of keeping the body well-nourished and healthy. In both cases, the key word is "sustainability."

Your ideal diet should not merely help you lose weight or feel good right now. It should also be sustainable in the long-term. Until recently, health care has been dominated by the use of powerful drugs that directly attack microbes, kill cancer cells, numb pain, and suppress inflammation. Yet, these same chemicals have a tendency to disrupt the internal environment, thus making us more vulnerable to disease, and therefore more dependent on these same toxic drugs.

The flaw in the above strategy is obvious. It makes no sense to remove the signs and symptoms of a disease, while neglecting its cause. It makes no sense to use therapies that make you feel better in the moment, but degrade your health in the long run.

Granted, there is value in being able to quickly remove a life-threatening infection, but it is likely to return if the cause of the infection (a weakened immune system) is not addressed. This was eventually recognized by Louis Pasteur, one of the earliest and strongest advocates of the germ theory.

For many years, Pasteur used to argue with his friend and colleague, Claude Bernard, as to the best way to rid the body of disease. Pasteur was in favor of attacking the pathogenic microbes, while Bernard insisted that the internal environment, which he called the inner "terrain" or "soil," was more important.

Obviously, Pasteur was the one who won out. Most school children eventually learn about Louis Pasteur. I remember first reading about him when I was in the fifth grade. In contrast, I did not learn of Claude Bernard until I entered chiropractic school. However, what most people do not realize is that Louis Pasteur had changed his mind, later in life. On his deathbed, he supposedly recanted, "Bernard was right. I was wrong. The microbe is nothing, the soil is everything."[2]

About 117 years after Pasteur uttered his dying words, and on the other side of the Atlantic Ocean, I found myself shopping at a local growers market. I stopped by one of the booths and examined the fresh corn on the cob, sitting on the counter. As usual, I asked the farmer if the corn had been sprayed. He gave me the usual answer: "You can't grow corn in these parts without pesticides."

As a rule, I buy organic or naturally grown produce, but since I enjoy corn on the cob in the summer, I sometimes compromise and buy conventionally grown corn. However, on that particular occasion, I decided to not purchase the corn. A few minutes later, I stopped by another booth, filled with produce from a local organic farm — including corn on the cob that looked exceptionally good. I asked the farmer if he used any sprays. He said no, so I bought some corn, took it home, and ate it.

The corn was amazingly delicious. It was perhaps, the best I have ever had. So, I returned to the same booth the following week, to get more. Once again, I was so impressed by the quality, that I felt compelled to inquire as to how they managed to grow such great-looking and great tasting corn, without pesticides and chemical fertilizers. The gentleman in the booth, a local grower who had been practicing organic farming for many years, responded, "It's all in the soil." I think that Claude Bernard would have agreed.

The body, and the food plants that feed the body, will both thrive when we focus less on killing the disease, and instead give more attention to nurturing the conditions that promote life. If the soil is neglected or mistreated, vitality diminishes. This is how the body becomes dependent on strong drugs, and food plants become dependent on pesticides and other toxic chemicals.

Rehabilitation of the soil is a long and arduous process. The farmer often does not have the time or money to make it feasible — just as most individuals do not have the time or knowledge to wean themselves off the antibiotics, antihistamines, pain medication, and stimulants. Both the farmer and the consumer are stuck on a treadmill of increased dependency on chemicals that gradually degrade the inner and outer soil.

With our personal health, we generally wait until conditions become intolerable, and then we take action. Hopefully the action takes the form of no longer doing the things that cause the problem, as we finally give our inner landscape the opportunity to rebuild itself. On the environmental side, happily, that time seems to have arrived. There seems to be a massive grassroots awakening to the simple facts that both our inner and outer soil must be treated with the same tender loving care.

Organic Farming and Beyond

The first step to healing the body and improving our methods of food production is to remember the famous words of Hippocrates: "Above all else, do no harm." He was referring to the practice of medicine, of course, but the same principle applies to food production. Regarding food production, doing no harm means growing food in a way that respects the integrity of the food and of the land. Simple enough. This is the basic strategy of organic farming. Beyond that, we also have to remember that there is an inherent difference in the environmental impact of producing the different food groups. Below is a brief description of how the production of each of these food groups impacts the environment.

Grains, Legumes, and Vegetables

Even before the days of synthetic herbicides, pesticides, and heavy farm machinery, intensive grain farming has historically turned fertile land into deserts. The very act of cutting down forests to make room for cultivated fields tends to dry up creeks and reduce local rainfall. As much as half the rain in a forest is generated by the forest itself.[3] When vast amounts of forest are cut down, there will be a dramatic reduction in the amount of moisture in the land, as well as triggering extremes in temperatures — hotter summers, colder winters, hotter days, colder nights. Intensely hot days and cold nights are typical of deserts.

The absence of underground root systems and resultant decrease in moisture, combined with frequent plowing of the field, result in the loss of topsoil and reduced fertility. This is how the central part of the United Sates was reduced to a dust bowl. It was the end result of many years of intensive grain farming. The same has occurred in other areas of the world, throughout history. The only difference is that now, we can destroy the land faster.

Vegetables have historically been more environmentally friendly than grains, simply because the former are grown in smaller quantities. The same applies to legumes, which provide the added benefit of adding nitrogen back into the soil.

In addition, legumes often have deeper roots, which allow them to bring up minerals from the subsoil.

Historically, some farmers have been mindful enough to "rotate" their crops, growing grains in a given area one year and legumes the next, thus mitigating the strain on the land. However, crop rotation does not reduce the degradation of the soil that results from plowing the land every year and compressing it with repeated traffic from farm animals and vehicles. This practice disrupts soil organisms and delicate root systems that normally help to maintain the fertility of the soil, and prevent erosion.

In light of the facts described above, why have grains dominated the food supply? The answer is that grains have historically been a great survival food. Grains were the singular commodity that allowed for the emergence of civilization as we know it.

However, civilization as we know it seems to be enmeshed with war, poverty, disease, and exploitation — all of which seem to be related to large-scale grain production. Fresh fruits and vegetables are not practical for feeding an army on the move, or a population of slaves working in mines, or constructing palaces.

The exploits of Julius Cesar, Alexander the Great, and other conquerors were made possible by grains and, to a lesser extent, dry beans. Meat, when available, was also helpful, but grains and dry beans were ideal for an army on the move, because these foods are light weight, pack a lot of calories, and can be stored indefinitely.[4] If meat was an option, the cows and goats could simply walk along with the troops until they were ready for slaughter.

History is filled with marauders and conquers from colder northern regions descending upon warmer southern regions. In colder regions, people typically lived on grains and beans, and to a lesser extent, meat and dairy. With these commodities, they were able to send their armies to plunder or subjugate populations in southern regions where fresh fruits and vegetables were plentiful, but armies were not. For example, the armies of the Roman Empire were invincible in Greece, the Mideast, and Africa. However, they were defeated (repeatedly) by armies from Northern Europe.

Animal Products

About 40% of the world's grain is used to raise livestock. This number is especially significant when we consider that much of the caloric value of the grains is lost when fed to farm animals. Specifically, it takes about 16 pounds of grains to produce one pound of beef. In terms of energy, it takes about 11 times as much fossil fuel to make one calorie of animal protein as it does to make one calorie of plant protein. Even if beef is grass-fed, the production of one pound of beef requires almost 20,000 liters of water, and ties up a lot of land that could otherwise be used to grow plant foods more efficiently.

At the present time, about 30% of available land is used for raising livestock. Of special concern is the rapid destruction of rain forests for conversion into pasture land, which has an adverse effect on climate, promoting extreme temperatures and desertification, even in areas far removed from the deforestation.[5] Another concern is that factory-farmed beef, pork, and poultry pose a major environmental hazard, especially in the contamination of ground water.

Fish, historically, have been the healthiest and most environmentally friendly of the flesh foods. However, since over-fishing is exceeding the capacity of the world's oceans and lakes, fish farming is becoming more common, which is not much better on the environment than factory farming of cows, pigs, and chickens.

Environmental Impact of Wheat and Meat
- Intensive grain farming turns fertile land into deserts.
- Loss of forests results in extremes in temperatures and desertification.
- Growing grains and raising food animals, especially the latter, on a massive scale, are the most expensive and least energy efficient ways of producing food. Both require heavy machinery that burn fossil fuel, and send poisonous petrochemicals into the soil, ground water, and air.
- Animal waste, herbicides, and pesticides from large factory farms are major polluters of ground water.
- The routine use of antibiotics in animal agriculture has contributed to the development of virulent bacteria, such as deadly strains of E. Coli.

Fruits, Nuts, and Seeds

All else being equal, these foods are typically the most environmentally friendly to produce, because they usually grow on trees and perennial bushes. Calorie for calorie, and acre for acre, these foods tend to have the greatest yield of all the food groups. In addition, they do not require annual replanting, so they are much less labor intensive, require far less fossil fuel, and the least amount of disturbance to the soil. By their very nature, trees help maintain and add to the fertility of the soil. The deep and extensive root systems minimize or eliminate the need for watering, as well as bringing up minerals from the subsoil.

Green is Clean

Beyond the purely nutritional considerations, if humans hypothetically used fruits and vegetables, and some nuts and seeds, as the primary source of calories, the environment would be transformed, becoming progressively greener and cleaner. Granted, we are speaking here of a diet resembling that of our primate relatives. Most individuals would find this impractical for one reason or another. Furthermore, in terms of food production, the use of these foods as the basis for human nutrition might seem unrealistic, because of their great bulk, weight, need for refrigeration, and perishability, all of which translate into significantly higher prices per calories. However, with your kind indulgence, I will add my own vision as to how this might be done.

Firstly, I am inclined to agree that the "greening" of the Earth is not a very practical idea — if we assume it must occur from the top down, through central planning. In other words, it will probably not occur through radical social and ecological engineering on a massive scale, through acts of Congress, the UN, or funding from mammoth corporations, but rather would happen with the most ease and grace if allowed to evolve slowly over time, as a natural consequence of more and more people simply choosing to eat more fresh produce, especially those food items that come from trees and perennial bushes.

In other words, it is not about legislation, it is about education. As our collective awareness evolves, it will compel a corresponding evolution of the political and economic forces — which ultimately must respond to what the consumer wants, otherwise, these institutions could not function for very long. As any student of the economy knows, the market will adjust itself to supply whatever the public wants.

In other words, the simplest and most harmonious way to change the market and change agriculture in the direction of healthier foods and healthier environment is to allow them to evolve *from the bottom up*, through the choices, actions, and enterprise of those same people who desire the foods in question.

This is not to suggest that large corporations and governments have no rightful place in this picture. I am simply suggesting that their natural role in this hypothetical transformation will become clear when they can just step aside and let it happen as a natural consequence of the collective will of the people — a will that can emerge as naturally and organically as that of a dependent child growing into a responsible adult.

Simply put, the rightful place of big corporations and central governments is established when all parties realize that the legitimate political power of governments, and financial power of corporations, are derived from the people they claim to serve — and to whom they are naturally accountable.

Bridging the Reality Gap

The above paragraph does not merely describe an abstract utopian ideal. It is a reality of politics and economics that is so simple and easy to grasp that it has been called "self-evident." Where do governments get their power? From we the people. Where do wealthy corporations get their wealth? From we the people. Who is ultimately responsible for legitimate governments and honest businesses being infiltrated by dictators and robber barons? We the people. We allow it when we stop paying attention. We allow it when we drug ourselves into a state of lethargy, apathy, and dependency. The wolves do not appear until the people turn into sheep.

Even those who want to be responsible citizens can eventually become frustrated and confused because their efforts to "think globally and act locally" seem to be mysteriously diverted in the opposite direction! In other words, we talk about building communities, and creating strong local economies, and sustainable food production, but we somehow find ourselves supporting politics that shifts the power away from communities and local governments, and into the hands of monolithic bureaucracies on the federal and even international levels — which have a tendency to not respond to the will of the people, but rather to the corporations with the most money.

Though we might try to cover the sense of apathy and futility with a veneer of positive thinking and optimism, we gradually start behaving like the slaves and serfs of olden times who gave up their hope for a better life and simply resigned themselves to their "fate."

We can see evidence of this secret sense of hopelessness as reactive sarcasm and cynicism in the general public. We see it even in a so-called "free society" that is willing to have a ring placed in its collective nose, passively submitting to the powers that be, even in the presence of blatant acts of injustice and corruption. We see the wrong, but feel helpless to do anything about it, so we tone down our capacity to feel, and turn our eyes away, simply as a matter of personal survival.

However, such apathy covers an even deeper desire for liberation, which is still very much alive, simply because it cannot die. No matter how long a slave remains a slave, the innate desire for freedom persists. It can only be drugged and sedated. It lies dormant, like a seed, waiting for the day it can awaken.

I am inclined to believe that we, in our collective human journey, have gathered the knowledge, and hopefully garnered the wisdom, to create (or re-create) the "garden" where fruit and peace are plentiful and readily available to anyone who sincerely desires them.

I do not merely speak hypothetically here. Such knowledge seems to be quietly taking root as innovative methods of food production, most notably, permaculture.

Permaculture

Permaculture might be the ultimate way to "think globally and act locally." Permaculture is a blend of tradition and modern science, utilizing the local climate, shape of the land, and natural water resources to maximize productivity, while maintaining and even enhancing the fertility of the soil. It encourages the growth of food-bearing plants that thrive best in a given environment, taking advantage of synergistic relationships between various species, and adjusting the work so it takes into account the natural ecological succession or "maturation" of land.

Once the permaculture system is allowed to reach maturity, it tends to continue on its own, with relatively little intervention by the stewards of the land. For example, the need for labor-intensive cultivation is greatly reduced, simply by maximizing the use of trees and perennial bushes that pretty much take care of themselves.

If the claims of its advocates are valid, permaculture might possibly be the most efficient and sustainable way of producing food, offering a greater yield than chemical farming, or traditional organic farming. Such systems are being used to turn empty lots and useless lawns into productive and esthetically appealing gardens.[6] Permaculture systems are quietly being established throughout the world, transforming barren land and deserts into lush gardens and orchards.

Though fruits, nuts, and seeds are the foods that can be grown most abundantly and efficiently in such a system, vegetables, grains, and traditional farm animals can also be integrated, so they add to the overall usefulness of the system, rather than depleting and polluting the environment.

Reasons to Favor Perennial Food Plants

- Compared to annual plants, most perennials grow taller and therefore have a greater yield per acre.
- Perennials tend to be heartier and have deeper roots, making them more resistant to drought and pestilence.
- Perennials do not require annual replanting and therefore are less labor intensive and less costly to maintain.
- Annual plants tend to degrade and compact the soil due to frequent cultivation and shallow roots, requiring the use of expensive (and toxic) chemicals to protect the plants and stimulate growth. In contrast, perennial plants tend to build soil.
- For all the reasons given above, perennials support small family-owned organic farms, which, in turn, translate into fresh, locally-produced food.

Contrast with Grain Farming

Compared to permaculture, intensive grain farming, even when done with traditional methods, requires a lot more time and energy. As a young child in Sicily, I got to see just how labor-intensive grain farming can be. I used to watch my father work his wheat field in the latter days of animal-power and pitchforks — circa 1959.

Like other farmers in the area, my father turned the soil with a one-blade plow, pulled by one or two mules. I thought it was the coolest thing to watch, and I never grew tired of it. However, I'm sure it got old real fast for my father, who, in addition to being a hard-working man, was also intelligent and was ever looking for more efficient and elegant ways of doing things. I suspect his innovative mind would have embraced permaculture principles if given the pertinent information, and had time to think it through.

However, such information was not available to him, and grain farming did not allow him enough leisure time to indulge the creative and visionary side of his nature. After he plowed his field, he had to plow it again. Then, he spread the seeds. Then, he hitched up his mules to a flat wooden board, which he stood upon, as the animals dragged it all over the field to press the seeds into the soil, so as to minimize loss from birds and other grain-eaters.

And still there was no rest. The harvest came quickly in early June and was equally labor intensive. It started with cutting the wheat stalks close to the ground with a small hand-held sickle. Then, my father and his helpers bound up the stalks into bales, which were carried to a small cleared area, centrally located in the wheat field, where the bales were unbound and arranged in a ring, thus setting the stage for the next step.

At this point, my father took his two mules to the perimeter of the ring of harvested wheat. Leaving the animals standing on the wheat, he walked to the center of the ring, still holding the reins. He then uttered the Sicilian version of "giddy-up," as the animals commenced trotting around the ring. Typically, he started singing a song, which I guess was intended to help the mules maintain their rhythm.

The mule-powered thrashing was, ideally, done on a windy day, because the next step was to throw the wheat stalks into the air with a pitch fork, causing the liberated wheat berries to fall almost straight to the ground, while the straw was blown several feet away.

And the process continued. Using a shovel, one person threw the wheat berries into a large sieve held by two people who shook it back and forth to separate the wheat berries from small rocks and other debris that had resisted the wind. Finally, the wheat was placed inside burlap bags, and taken to storage until it was sold or bartered for other goods, or taken to the local mill to be ground up into flour for our family's use.

At that point, my father's job (in wheat production, at least) was complete, and my mother's task began. She was in charge of converting the flour into our daily bread and pasta. Placing a large amount of flour on a square wooden board, she made a crater in the middle of the pile and filled it with warm water. Yeast was also added, unless the dough was to be used to make pasta. She then mixed the flour with her hands (which looked like great fun to my young eyes), until it became a cohesive mass of dough, which she then kneaded for quite a while. When that task was finally complete, the dough was either converted into pasta, or allowed to rise if it was to become bread.

Eventually, the risen dough was cut and shaped into individual spherical loaves, which were allowed to rise a second time, during which they settled into their characteristic saucer shape. While the loaves were rising, my mother had to fire up her stone-and-mortar igloo oven. Her fuel consisted of twigs, hay, and anything else that burned. She had to collect her fuel each time she baked bread, because there was no convenient pile of wood or coal next to the oven. Coal was too expensive for this purpose, and large pieces of wood were rather scarce because most of the trees had been cut down long ago.

The hay and twigs were stuffed into the oven and ignited, with the help of bits of sulfur from our local volcano. My mother had to tend the fire continuously with a long metal poker, frequently feeding it, because straw and twigs burn quickly. As my mother carried out her task, heat and smoke emerged from the arched doorway on the side of the oven, where she stood with her metal poker.

After the oven was sufficiently heated, the ashes were removed, and the hot oven floor swept and washed clean, filling the oven with steam. The risen loaves were then individually placed in the oven, and the doorway covered with a flat piece of iron or slate, its edges sealed with a black paste made of ashes removed from the oven.

After about 45 minutes, she unsealed the oven door and checked the bread. If it felt ready, she removed all the loaves. If not, she gave them more time, because the oven was still plenty hot.

Imagine doing this during the long and hot Sicilian summers. Sicily is not that far from Africa, and is often visited by an intensely hot and dry wind from the Sahara Desert. Imagine doing this 3 or 4 days per week, during the busiest time of the year, because she did not merely have to bake enough bread for her husband and seven growing children, but also the field workers, hired by my father. Not surprisingly, when she finally came to America, she said, "Never again" and refused to bake any more bread for the rest of her life.

Historical Perspective

While my father grew the wheat, and my mother transformed it into bread and pasta, they probably did not realize they were teaching me history in a manner more real and palpable than anything I could have gotten from a book or class. Years later, as an avid student of history, I eventually learned that my parents' wheat-farming and bread-making routine was virtually the same as that of their predecessors in past centuries, throughout Europe and other parts of the world.

Imagine, how it might have been in the past, when peasants had to do what my parents did (and then some!), so as to provide enough bread (sometimes all of it) for the nobility and their servants and armies — for which the peasants frequently did not get paid, for this was how they were "taxed."

The peasants often did not even own their farms, and if they did, it would not have made much difference. They were de facto slaves to the land. They were serfs who had resigned themselves to their fate, just as the nobility took it for granted they were divinely ordained to rule the peasants, who were seen as inferior beings. The elite looked upon the peasants with disdain, or perhaps pity, but ultimately they were commodities, like horses, cows, and sheep.

I am reminded that in my hometown and surrounding areas, during the time of my childhood, individuals who had somehow "risen above" the need to work the land, sometimes looked down on those who still had to do so. This was probably a residue from the attitude of the aristocracy of past centuries, who basically lived parasitically on the peasants, while often holding them in contempt.

However, I'm not implying that the nobles of olden times were all cruel and callous slave drivers. They were simply a product of their time. Marie Antoinette, queen of France and wife of Louis the XVI, supposedly was once told that the peasants were complaining because they had no bread to eat. She allegedly replied, "Let them eat cake." The "cake" was not what we call cake, as in a birthday cake, but rather referred to the hard crusty material that gets caked on the outside of the oven, from repeated exposure to steam and flour dust — which I also seem to remember from my mother's igloo oven.

Marie Antoinette's apparently taunting attitude is said to have spurred the French Revolution. However, the words she supposedly spoke, and their implied callousness, is seriously questioned by historians, because it did not fit her personality — as suggested in her later biography: "It is quite certain that in seeing the people who treat us so well despite their own misfortune, we are more obliged than ever to work hard for their happiness. The King seems to understand this truth."[7]

Apparently, the "Let them eat cake" story was cooked up later to add fuel to the French Revolution. If anything, Marie Antoinette, and many of the nobility of the day, were not totally insensitive to the needs of the peasants. More likely, they were extravagant and frivolous due to their sheltered lives.

I mention all this, because we can see a similar frivolousness and extravagance today in developed countries. As with nobility of old, living in their castles, we are far removed from the violence, poverty, and other hardships of those living in politically and economically unstable regions. These people, trapped in poverty, are often the same ones who provide the cheap labor that provide the rest of us with the food and manufactured goods that help maintain our standard of living.

For those of us who lead a relatively sheltered life, it is easy to be indifferent to and even condone gross exploitation. However, it is another matter entirely if we see what is actually happening to support our lifestyle. Our sleeping conscience tends to awaken when we finally look into the eyes of those who suffer and sometimes die, so that we can prosper and maintain our opulent lifestyle. Most individuals would respond with concern and a genuine desire to right the wrong, as did Marie Antoinette.

In stark contrast to the aristocracy of Old Europe, the founders of the United States of America, including George Washington and Thomas Jefferson, considered farming to be the noblest of professions, vital to the new nation. Their enthusiastic support of agriculture is reflected in the Constitution, which, until the early 20th century, had allowed small family-owned farms to thrive and prosper.

What went wrong? Part of the issue is the fact that the United States, like most other developed nations, has relied heavily on labor-intensive grain farming and large-scale animal agriculture. Both seem to carry the very seeds of exploitation and degradation, regardless of the political system.

Alternate History

What if permaculture had played a more central role in the rise of civilization? I suspect history might have unfolded differently. Perhaps famine would have been rare, because these systems are locally supported, locally maintained, and are largely self-sustaining and resistant to drought and pestilence. Perhaps some of the "useless" land around the world would not be so useless.

What if half the wheat fields and pasture land in the world were allowed to mature into stable food forests and ecological gardens? What if some of the annual crops that dominate our food supply were replaced with productive trees and other perennials? Theoretically, the endless cycles of annual plowing, replanting, and weeding would be drastically reduced. With perennial food plants, the harvest is the most labor intensive phase of food production, after which there is little else to do, because most of the food is ready to eat with little or no processing — no need for thrashing, milling, mixing, kneading, and baking. In other words, workload is reduced and yield increased, simply by cooperating with Nature, rather than trying to conquer it.

According to the claims of those knowledgeable in the field, the widespread use of permaculture principles could result in the production of more than enough food to supply every man, woman, and child on the planet. The only real limitation of such systems is that they are not very conducive to greed, exploitation, and war.

What about the "Peasants?"

A little closer to home for me, I imagine things might have been different in my hometown in Sicily, where the rare orchard seemed like an oasis in a desert of wheat fields. During my childhood, my grandfather was only one of three individuals in the entire region who made a living growing fruits and vegetables, rather than wheat.

On the other hand, if permaculture had been the preferred method of food production, my grandfather's huge garden might have been the rule rather than the exception. Even relatively dry farm land, such as my father's old wheat field, could have supported such a system, if intelligently managed with simple techniques for harvesting natural sources of water. My father may have had more time to play his mandolin and write poetry — which he finally did in his later years. And my mother may have had the opportunity to continue her education beyond grade school, to develop her sharp mathematical mind.

I share all this, not to lament the past, but rather to invite an expanded vision of what is possible for the future. It is natural to respectfully recognize the hard work, sacrifice, and mistakes of those who preceded us, for this is how we complete the past, learn from it, and move on, rather than mindlessly repeating the mistakes of our ancestors. For example, a close examination of history shows that permaculture systems are not new. They have been used throughout the world, since antiquity. They were apparently quite successful, but were largely forgotten.

Rebirth of Permaculture

In the Americas, we see evidence of humans encouraging the growth of stable food forests — centuries ago, before the arrival of the European explorers and conquerors. In fact, anthropologists visiting indigenous tribes in Africa, Asia, and South America, often did not realize that some of the surrounding "jungle" was actually a productive food forest, created by the locals.[8] However, after the indigenous people became "modernized," most of their food forests were replaced by conventional agriculture. The result? The one time self-sustaining natives became dependent on chemical fertilizers, pesticides, imported processed foods, and other modern conveniences, making them more vulnerable to drought, famine, poverty, and disease. Much of the poverty in so-called third world countries did not exist until they were influenced by developed nations.

Currently, the oldest known food forest is a man-made oasis in Morocco, which supposedly once fed an entire village. It is said to be about 2000 years old — and was still functional at the time of this writing.[9] Such systems apparently have been even more common in the Far East, such as a reportedly 300 year old food forest in Vietnam.[10]

The Tao of Permaculture

The greater use of permaculture principles in Asia is not surprising, because it bears a striking resemblance to Taoism, which is practiced widely in the East. Taoism consists of principles and techniques for promoting vibrant health and harmonious relationship with the life around us. Permaculture uses essentially the same core principles and applies them to food production. The table below compares the principles of permaculture with those of traditional Taoism.

Principles	Taoism	Permaculture
Observe and Conserve	To promote health and longevity, conserve energy. To conserve energy, observe and follow the cycles and rhythms of Nature.	Observe and learn as much as you can about a given system, so you can get the best yield with the least amount of work.
Patience	The best way to fight a battle is to not fight it at all.[11] Hurrying waists energy and slows down progress.	Systems that that reach maturity at their own pace are the most stable and productive. Don't rush progress with chemicals.
Relationship	The key to health and longevity is the relationship of the body parts.	The key to a stable ecological system is the dynamic relationship of all parts, not the role of any one component.
Opposites	The dance of Yin and Yang allows for energy flow and creation.	The most productivity occurs at the boundary of two different systems or environments, such as the interface between a wooded area and meadow.
Harmony	When Yin and Yang are in harmony, they complement each other.	Arrange all elements so they complement one another. For example, corn provides a climbing pole for beans, which provide nitrogen for the corn.
Obstacles into Assets	The best way to defeat enemies is to change them into friends.[12]	Rather than fighting weeds, find ways of using them to build soil, provide food, and create habitat.

Here is an excerpt from *Gaia's Garden*, by Toby Hemenway, describing the transformation of New Mexico desert land:

"...I stepped out of my car and was blasted by the mid-90s heat and searing glare reflected from the bare, eroded hillsides nearby. But before me was a wall of greenery, a lush landscape that I had spotted from at least a mile away, in soothing contrast to the yellow sand and gravel of the desert.

"I entered the garden through a gap between arching trees, and the temperature plummeted. The air here was fresh, cool and moist, unlike the dusty sinus withering stuff I'd been breathing outside. A canopy of walnut trees, pinion pine and New Mexico black locust sheltered a lush understory of pomegranates, nectarines, jujube trees, and almonds. An edible passionflower swarmed up a rocky wall. Grapevines arched over an entry trellis. Two small ponds sparkled with rainwater caught by the adobe roof. Winking brightly from under shrubs and along pathways were endless varieties of flowers, both native and exotic.

"...They blended berry bushes and small fruit trees into an edible hedge along the north border, to offer them food as well as block the winds that roared down the nearby canyon. All these techniques combined into a many-pronged strategy to build fertile soil, cast shade, dampen the wild temperature swings of the desert, and conserve water. Together these practices create a mild, supportive place to grow a garden. Slowly the barren landscape transformed into a young, multistoried food forest.

"Roxanne carried pruning shears as she walked and lopped off the occasional too-exuberant branch from the mulberries, plums, black locusts, and other vigorously growing trees and shrubs that lined the paths. These would feed her turkeys or become more mulch.

"Roxanne and her helpers had rejuvenated a battered plot of desert, created a thick layer of rich soil, and brought immense biodiversity to a once impoverished place. Here in the high desert was almost too much water and shade. Food was dropping from the trees faster than they could harvest, and birds that no one had seen for years were making a home in the yard."[13]

Support your local small family farm

The lush garden described above was created in a climate that was hotter and drier than the wheat fields in my hometown. There is an obvious and powerful message here: If we can create a lush garden in a hot and dry desert, we can do it just about anywhere.

I also find it significant that such systems do not depend on controls from a large central government or funding from huge corporations. Such systems can evolve easily and gracefully controlled entirely by the local community, and empowered totally by the hard work and ingenuity of individuals, whose primary motivation is simply to provide a good home, good food, and a good life for their families.

Until permaculture becomes well established, individuals who wish to "vote with their money" can support organic farms (or any farm that favors sustainable methods of food production). In fact, as permaculture principles become more widely known, small family owned farms will have a better chance of succeeding because they will become more economically feasible.

What will allow this vision to become reality? Your financial support. Make it your business to buy some of your food from such farms, and they will grow and prosper.

Looking at the bigger picture, I believe that a nation of educated consumers is the most powerful force for changing how governments govern, and how businesses take care of business. Voting with your money is still the most effective way to influence the evolution of government and business — especially with regard to food production. When enough consumers make it known they are paying attention to the quality of food and the ethical side of eating, the food producers will also pay attention.

At this point, another reality check is in order. Other authors have already voiced the ideas described above. Attempts to implement them have repeatedly broken down. For example, as previously mentioned, permaculture systems had been used in the past, and were abandoned. Why did they fizzle out, and give way to labor-intensive and land-eroding agriculture? It is a complex issue, but it does have an underlying simplicity, which, I think, can be nicely summarized with just one word — maturity

In order for permaculture to work, we must allow the land to reach ecological maturity. However, in order for us to do that, we must also do our homework. Yes, permaculture allows us to do much less physical work — provided we first do our mental work. Permaculture requires us to study the land and the plants. Permaculture compels us to cultivate patience and slow down, so we can notice pertinent details. It compels us to expand our vision to be able to see the intimate relationship between all living things — not just as a philosophical ideal, but also in specific ways that are immediately applicable to the needs of the day. In its own subtle way, permaculture encourages us to shift from competition to cooperation, from conquest to collaboration.

In other words, we can allow the land to reach ecological maturity only if *we* are ready to reach maturity — which brings us to the next section.

Spiritual and Humane Considerations

The spiritual side of eating has to do with adjusting food intake so as to support our relationship with the fundamental forces that create the universe. The humane side of eating, in the broadest sense, has to do with acknowledging our relationship with the life around us. We see this most obviously in the practice of ethical vegetarianism or veganism, which refrain from killing or exploiting animals, and typically include a similar regard for other humans affected by our food choices.

Naturally, we do not have to adhere to any sort of religious or spiritual system in order to be mindful of the humane aspects of eating. However, I address these two topics under the same heading because the two seem too closely connected to justify putting them in two totally different boxes.

Firstly, both have to do with relationship. The spiritual aspirant asks the question, "Will this food help or hinder my relationship with the God?" The humane eater asks the question, "When I nourish my body and experience the sensuous pleasure of this meal, who pays the price?" To fully appreciate just how deeply connected these two questions are, let us first give each one some thoughtful attention.

Our Relationship with the Source

If your food choices are a personal matter, your spiritual life is even more so. You are the only person on this Earth who has the natural authority to choose how you will nourish your soul, just as you are the only one who chooses how to nourish your body. Therefore, I offer the following ideas in the same manner in which I present the purely nutritional information — with the understanding that *you* decide how these ideas pertain to you, if at all.

Dietary injunctions or guidelines among the various religions are more the rule than the exception. This alone suggests there is some kind of interface between diet and spiritual cultivation. Looking a bit deeper, the dietary choices often involve a belief that all living things are ultimately united.

This interconnectedness is often described by mystics as the awareness that we are *related* to all living things around us, simply because we stem from a common source. For example, Christian traditions describe the creative source as the "Heavenly Father," which obviously makes all humans brothers and sisters.

Granted, we might feel the connection most strongly with those to whom we are genetically or culturally closest, but ultimately, as the story goes, we are all branches of the same tree of life, and somewhere deep inside, we know it.

Deepening ones spiritual experience essentially translates into "shifting" one's position on the tree of life to progressively larger branches, until finally we find ourselves on the main trunk, which means our sense of kinship with *all* life becomes as palpable as our sense of kinship with our biological siblings.

This is when we might experience something resembling the writings of Saint Francis of Assisi, whose connection with God reportedly became so deep that he regarded everything in the created universe as his brother or sister, including the sun and the moon.[15]

As the spiritual cultivation deepens further, we eventually get to the very "root" of our spiritual existence, which means we do not merely feel related to others — we might actually feel compelled to declare, "I *am* the other!" This sentiment has been expressed in various ways, such as Jesus supposedly saying, "What you do to the least of your brethren, you do to me."

Our deepest connection with the creator of all life might be beyond human understanding, but it also shows up in some very tangible ways that are essential to survival, such as expressions of genuine kindness, generosity, thankfulness, and a natural inclination to do no harm. These are not merely abstract ideals. They are the pearls of great price that make life worth living — without which society breaks down. I suspect that our ancestors in the ancient world were keenly aware of this.

The food connection

How might food influence this process of navigating from the peripheral branches to the main trunk of the tree of life? That depends. The use of food to further spiritual development is common in the old religions. On the other hand, what is less obvious is that our attitude toward those very same food choices might actually work *against* spiritual cultivation.

On the positive side, here are some nutritional and physiological reasons to believe that the old religions were on to something:

- Religion, at its best, is about providing a way of directing emotional energy into spiritual awareness, which, in everyday life, typically shows up as an attitude of good will and trust. Foods made of animal flesh are likely to contain stress hormones, such as cortisol, as well as stimulating higher levels of testosterone, both of which can drive our emotional energy the other way — into survival mode. High levels of cortisol and testosterone in the body are likely to make us feel more competitive, aggressive, suspicious, and fearful.
- Animal flesh, such as red meat, is high in uric acid, as well as encouraging uric acid production in the body. Uric acid affects the body in a manner similar to caffeine — it stimulates cortisol production.
- Fruits and vegetables often contain phytonutrients that positively influence brain chemistry. For example, some flavonoids favor higher levels

of serotonin, which is then used to make melatonin and other substances associated with calmness and feelings of loving kindness toward others — in essence, countering the emotional effects of the stress hormones.
- A plant-based diet might support spiritual cultivation in a similar manner to fasting.[16,17]

On the Other Hand…

When I think of individuals I've known personally over the years who have embodied spiritual values, kindness, and thoughtfulness, the first ten or so who come to mind were not vegetarians. I have also known vegetarians and vegans who were chronically depressed, easily angered, and not very tolerant.

Some non-vegetarians might be quick to suggest that such behavior is due to imbalances produced by modern vegetarian and vegan diets that feature large amounts of refined grains, refined sugar, highly processed soy products, and a lack of omega-3 oils. This might be valid in some instances. However, beyond the purely nutritional considerations, I have also gotten the impression that vegetarianism can insidiously degenerate into yet another way of drifting into an "us-and-them" mentality and provoking conflict — which means it is hurting, not helping, spiritual cultivation.

The right kind of plant based diet can, indeed, support spiritual cultivation. On the other hand, to the extent we use our "clean diet" as a badge of honor to exalt ourselves over others; we sicken the heart and add to our sense of isolation. In essence, such an attitude keeps us exiled on the peripheral branches of the tree of life — where all beings are separate, and often hostile toward each other.

I am reminded here of when I first started to explore a vegetarian diet many years ago. I was doing so strictly for health reasons, but I was also aware of many individuals doing it for spiritual, humane, or environmental reasons. Some of them did it lightheartedly, while others seemed to have an ax to grind, insisting or implying that eating animal flesh was only for those who were spiritually dense and socially uninformed. Without realizing it, I was gradually absorbing this attitude. Fortunately, while I was preparing a tasty vegetarian dinner, a sentence formed in my mind that abruptly ended my silent strutting about, and forever altered my course of thinking on this subject. The words were clear and distinct, as if a voice (and a jovial one at that) was speaking them into my ear. The message was, "No one is further from heaven than an arrogant vegetarian." I paused for a moment, and then burst out laughing.

Several years prior to that, I had received a similar message. I was still in my early years of attempting to eat a cleaner diet (again, for purely health reasons), which included a steady decrease in my use of animal products and all things fried and greasy. During that time, I was in the midst of ending a close relationship with a woman I had been dating, and found myself in my apartment, moping and feeling sorry for myself. Not surprisingly, I felt like eating something rich and heavy, even though I wasn't particularly hungry. At first, I resisted, but eventually decided to give in to my desire. So, I went to the local fast food restaurant for some chicken nuggets.

Once I got there, I experienced the old split again. I was looking forward to eating the chicken nuggets, even as I silently judged my choice as "unhealthy." I then looked around and proceeded to judge the other folks in the restaurant in the same manner. The judgment was barely noticeable. I would have forgotten it immediately if it weren't for a gentle wake-up call. Sitting at a table, I looked up. Directly in front of me, perhaps twenty feet away, a man and woman had just sat down, and were having a quiet conversation. That's when the miracle happened. As I looked at them, they stopped talking. Bowing their heads, they brought their hands together and gave prayerful thanks for their food. My mind stopped in its tracks, and experienced several seconds of blessed stillness. The first thought that emerged from the inner silence was "Thank you."

Our Relationship with Other Humans

Even if our sense of kinship with the other branches of the tree of life isn't as visceral and palpable as that of St. Francis, it still manages to reach the surface of our minds. It might show up as a feeling that has no words. Or it might show up more specifically as a knowing that any act of violence against others is violence against oneself; any deception of others is self-deception; stealing from others makes one poorer.

Even those who are adamantly agnostic might eventually get quiet enough to hear the voice of their own conscience, asking, "How do my food choices affect other humans? Was that coffee grown by farmers and workers who got a fair compensation for their honest work? Who is paying the price for the cheap 5-pound bag of sugar I buy at the supermarket? Who is paying the price for the inexpensive chocolate I eat? Is it cheap because it is grown on plantations in the Ivory Coast that use forced child labor?"[18] Even if the pragmatic mind doesn't quite understand why we would entertain such concerns, our conscience still haunts us.

Individuals who care about the poverty and famine in third world countries might be shocked to learn that these same cultures had no problem feeding, clothing, and sheltering themselves before they were influenced by industrialized nations.[8] The poverty in Haiti is one such example:

> "The largest portions of Haiti's best lands produce crops for export… With most of the very best land out of production for local food crops (beans, rice, and corn), the masses of people do not have access to land to grow food for eating or selling on the local market. Ironically, Haiti, a primarily agricultural land, is a net importer of food. At first one might think that this is not such a bad thing. After all, by selling crops on the international market, income is generated for Haiti, jobs are produced, and money circulates. Unfortunately none of this happens in any positive way for the great masses of people. First, these lands, which produce the export crops, are controlled by the elite of Haiti. Most of the imported cash goes to these owners/controllers of the land and most of it is not spent in Haiti, but in the more interesting markets of the United States and Europe. Not even a trickledown effect is felt from this flow of cash. Further, the farm wages are among the lowest in Haiti. Cane cutters spend an entire day in backbreaking work to cut a ton of sugar cane. For this long day one can expect $1.00 a day OR LESS!"[19]

Our Relationship with other Animals

Is it possible to be an ethical omnivore? Many vegans say no. My personal answer is yes. However, the reality of it might be too complicated for a black and white answer. As with other spiritual concerns, this is where we would do well to loosen our tight grip on our cherished belief systems, so we can listen to our hearts, and learn from each other.

Traditional hunting societies often recognize the presence of an intelligent being within the hunted animal. They recognize a being having the capacity to experience fear, pain, sorrow, and joy — a being no less deserving of respect and kindness than any human.

Naturally, if such sensibilities coexist with a desire to eat the same animal, inner conflict can easily arise. That contradiction could not be ignored by hunting societies that placed great value on an active spiritual life. Therefore, it is not surprising that so many hunting societies have a tradition of thanking or otherwise acknowledging the "spirit" in the animal. Similar sensibilities are seen in other cultures, as in the kosher laws of Judaism, which provide for the special treatment of food derived from animal sources.

The major religions of the Far East go one step further by advocating vegetarianism. Some of these old religions did eventually allow for the option of consuming animal flesh, but in their original version, all were strictly vegetarian and, in the case of Jainism, strictly vegan. Furthermore, some scholars suggest the three major religions of the West (Judaism, Christianity, and Islam) may also have had vegetarian origins. For example, the original Franciscan monastic order is said to have been vegetarian, as was its founder, St. Francis.[20]

On the Other Hand...

Historically, vegetarianism and veganism in the Eastern religions have often been linked with the belief in reincarnation and karma, and were rooted in the belief that we should practice compassion toward all beings. In contrast, the Western religions seemed to have abandoned the belief in reincarnation, just as they abandoned vegetarianism.

As vegetarianism in Western religions was "down-regulated," into specific dietary injunctions, the concept of karma was also simplified into the familiar Biblical concept of "sowing and reaping." In both Eastern and Western theology, the concept is essentially the same — we cannot escape the consequences of our own actions. Sooner or later, the scales will balance. Whatever we do unto life, life will do unto us.

However, in Eastern religions, the doctrine of karma is often applied mindlessly, resulting in a rigid interpretation of the law, which leads to misunderstanding and conflict, rather than inspiring compassion for all. For example, a close examination of the principle of reincarnation leads us to the obvious conclusion that the two parties in any conflicted relationship are working out their respective karma, which means their treatment of each other has to ultimately be balanced out. Any perception of exploitation is just that — a perception. It is but a momentary ripple in the great ocean of space-time. This does not mean we deny the feelings of anger or sadness at the perceived injustice or cruelty. It simply means we are willing to see the bigger picture.

It is easy to get angry or self-righteous when we see only part of any story, but when we remember that our human sight has its limits, we tend to be not so quick to anger, or to try to convert others to our way of thinking. We find it easier to give thoughtful consideration to both sides of any argument, rather than being blindly pulled into it, and adding to the drama.

That Could Be Me

For sure, we can still passionately speak out for those who cannot speak for themselves. We can still fight the good fight, when we feel the cause is just. The difference is that we tend to carry out our campaign from a different vantage point, one of greater calmness and, in my opinion, greater effectiveness.

Our awareness of the bigger picture does not have to be transcendental or unworldly. More typically it shows up as kindness or patience — simple, soft-spoken, and unpretentious. One way we know that compassion is real is when it is extended equally to the perceived villain and victim. Such compassion is simply the voice that says, "That could me."

Compassion is the ability to recognize that I could very well be the villain or the victim, given the right set of circumstances. This does not require spiritual training of any kind, but the simple willing to be honest with oneself. This is the compassion taught by such spiritual giants as Jesus Christ and the Buddha.

Do We Need to Eat Animal Flesh?

For most modern humans, the question of the morality of eating animal flesh never arises. Those who do ponder the issue typically conclude they require animal food to maintain their health. I personally am not in a position to refute this claim; therefore, I choose to err on the side of caution by allowing for the very real possibility that they are accurate in their assessment — in which case, I certainly would not deny them the same right I would extend to an eagle or a cat.

Admittedly, my attitude about this issue might reflect my own personal history. As a young child living in an agricultural community, I was exposed to the attitude that *all* animals are commodities. I was not encouraged to have pets. Dogs were for protection and herding sheep. Cats were for controlling the population of grain-eating rodents. Cows, pigs, and chickens were livestock.

Nonetheless, somewhere deep inside, I was affected by the obvious fact that livestock was, after all, *alive*. And, even though I did not contemplate the sentience of other animals, I did respond to it emotionally. As a child, I was fascinated by the sight of a wheat field being plowed, or my grandfather's garden being watered through its intricate system of irrigation canals. In contrast, I was repulsed by the sight of a chicken having its neck broken. One of the most disturbing sights of my early childhood was that of a pig being slaughtered outdoors. And yet, I did eat and enjoy chicken and pork. It was a simple matter of temporarily suppressing the unpleasant memory of having watched the same animal being slaughtered, just a few hours earlier.

I suppose I would have eventually become hardened to these realities of farm life, if I had stayed in my hometown, and become a farmer or sheepherder. However, it was not any easier several years later, as an adolescent living in In Brooklyn, NY, where my mother often asked me go buy our dinner at the live-chicken market.

Granted, I intellectually accepted the killing of animals for food as a reality of life. Even when I began to phase out animal products from my diet, it was for health reasons. However, the deeper feeling part of me was quietly thankful to be able to nourish my body adequately (indeed, optimally) without the need to kill or exploit animals.

Driving Your Own Car

I say all this to underscore my previous point of choosing to adjust my own diet and sense of ethics from within, which, as far as I can tell, requires that I refrain from imposing my own nutritional and ethical values on others. Over the years, I have gotten the impression that in order for me to really access my inner guidance, and calibrate my own moral compass, I have to be willing to allow others to do the same.

This is not to invalidate the message of ethical veganism. On the contrary, I believe such a message is one that needs to be heard, because, as various spiritual leaders and philosophers have pointed out, the manner in which we treat animals affects our own moral fiber, and eventually influences how we treat each other. However, I also believe this same vital message is weakened when delivered with too much urgency or harshness. We squeeze the life out of it by clutching it too tightly. I believe the message of ethical veganism will have its greatest impact if the persons delivering it are mindful that they are venturing into an area that is as emotionally sensitive as a person's relationship with his or her mother.

In my opinion, the message of ethical veganism will be best heard when the persons delivering it are willing to look at themselves, even as they hope the meat-eaters look at themselves. I speak here of an attitude that allows vegetarians and vegans to relate to meat-eaters in a manner that is free of the subtle (and perhaps unconscious) holier-than-thou attitude. I speak here of an attitude rooted in the perception of equality, communicated silently as the warmth of our shared humanity. This is how the often touchy subject of the following section can be discussed respectfully and with proper understanding.

We All Eat Living Things

As I see it, diet and spiritual cultivation must eventually converge for the simple reason that we all eat living things. When and how they converge is a private matter, but converge they must. Why? Quite simply, spiritual cultivation has to do with a recognition of the common origin of all life forms — including the life forms we happen to use as food. Regardless of which diet we chose, every time we eat, we are "communing" with life. Depending on how we do so, the event can enhance or diminish our deeper communion with the creative source of all life.

If the ancient Hindu idea of karma has any truth to it, that communion is very much a two way street. Regarding food, the nourishment, blessings, and harm travel in both directions. Beyond that simplistic model, the communion might have levels of subtlety that we cannot begin to touch with our human understanding.

However, before you even begin to explore that mysterious communion, you might be able to simplify things by first asking a more fundamental question: Do I really need to think about this stuff right now? As previously mentioned, *you* are in charge of establishing your priorities.

Yes, respect for the life and dignity of others (humans and animals) seems to be part of our natural spiritual development. However, when and how the individual answers that call is a very personal matter. I am inclined to think that our deeper relationship to the living things we use as food will be addressed with the most ease and grace if allowed to emerge from within, and in accordance with the cycles and seasons of the individual's life. On the other hand, the same issue becomes vexing and confusing when forced upon us through rigid doctrine or social pressure.

In other words, if the above narrative seems like abstract mind-gymnastics with no practical value for you, it probably is. When the question regarding your deeper relationship with food is allowed to emerge naturally from within, you can then give it thoughtful consideration. This is when you can truly contemplate the sentience of the beef cow, or for that matter, the carrot or apple.

The Old Carob Tree

Animals with a brain similar to ours seem to experience emotions similar to ours. They want to survive, just as we do. But, what about plants? Some studies suggest that plants may have a consciousness of sorts — different from ours, but supposedly similar enough to allow them to respond to us in ways that we might be tempted to interpret as happiness, sadness, and fear.[21]

I am reminded here of a carob tree on the outskirts of my hometown, during my early childhood. Its generous sprawling branches also provided a wonderful shade during the hot Sicilian summers, as one of my brother and I sat against its massive trunk, in the stillness and quiet of the afternoon. Our cows grazed in the field in front of us, against a background of rolling hills and mountains, as we ate bread and olives, or maybe some carob pods.

The tree was also a gathering place for many other youngsters. The very size and shape of the tree invited us to climb, play, and enjoy the carob bounty. Some of the peripheral branches hung straight down and approached the ground. They were thin enough to be very flexible but still strong enough for us to swing on. Its main branches diverged from the trunk at a point fairly close to the ground, making the tree very climbable. If I remember correctly, the point of divergence of its main branches from the trunk included a basin-like curved surface, where we could recline comfortably, and even take a nap.

Fifty-one years have passed since I used to play and relax under that tree. I guess I loved it, and in retrospect, I sometimes rather fancy that it loved me back. Some years ago, as an adult living in the United States, I once had a dream in which the tree had been cut down, which saddened me (in the dream). Surprisingly, I later found out that it had, indeed, been cut down — right around the time I had the dream! A coincidence? Perhaps. Are trees sentient beings? I cannot say for sure, but I'm inclined to think so.

Chapter 14
Summary and Final Musings

The introduction to this book offers two guidelines for healthy eating.
- Eat what your instincts tell you to eat.
- Eat generous amounts of fresh fruits and vegetables.

Chapters 1 through 10 provide the details. Most of those details are essentially the same as those in other books on nutrition and diet. My goal has been to present them in a way that guides you back to the simplicity of eating foods that both taste good and promote vibrant health.

The two guidelines stated above work very well together. They might be said to be synergistic. Specifically, consuming a generous amount of fresh fruits and vegetables supports instinctual eating. Likewise, in my experience, as we reawaken our food instincts, we are more likely to spontaneously favor fresh and minimally processed fruits and vegetables.

However, the above paragraph should not be taken to mean that I advocate a diet consisting totally or mostly of fruits and vegetables for everyone. I am simply adding my voice to the many others who point out that unprocessed fruits and vegetables are Nature's original "health food."

How much of these health foods should you consume? *You* are, ultimately, the best judge that. This book simply provides a map for reaching your personal "zone" of optimal eating. The last two sections of chapter 9 ("Fruit as a Staple Food," and "How to Invite More Fruits and Vegetables into Your Life") guide the reader through that process.

Fruit Is Not a Panacea

Since I strongly endorse fruit as a staple food, I wish to emphasize that its blessings depend on proper use, which varies from person to person. Using food as a staple food means you consume enough of it to fulfill a significant percentage (10% or more) of your caloric needs, as described in chapter 9. Some individuals may need to use it in modest amounts, while others can apparently thrive on a high-fruit diet. This is where I encourage you to use your educated common sense and instincts to determine what is appropriate for you. In other words, regardless of how you answer the question, "What should I eat," remember that the answer comes from within.

For those who do feel inclined to explore the possibility of increasing fruit consumption, here is a review of the main points to consider:

- Quality becomes increasingly important as your fruit consumption increases.
- The fruit we buy is the store is different from the fruits our ancestors ate. Though fruit quality and selection is likely to increase as the demand increases, we must still remember that store-bought fruit is probably hybridized, which may or not necessarily be a bad thing, depending on the fruit, but either way, it was also probably grown in less than ideal conditions, and was probably picked unripe. All this translates into a reduction of overall nutritional value, especially the mineral content.
- Even if fruit quality is very good, some individuals may simply be constitutionally unsuited for a high-fruit diet. Others may need to give the body time to gradually cleanse and rebalance itself, before it can efficiently process larger amounts of fruit. Yes, humans are, first and foremost, primates. And yes, primates are fundamentally designed to get the bulk of daily calories from fruit. However, we have been exiled from the tropical gardens of our ancestors, and have utilized non-primate foods long enough to approach a high-fruit diet with caution.
- High quality fruit is good food, but makes for a very poor drug. It cannot stimulate or sedate us, as do many of the cooked and heavily spiced foods. Neither can fruit provide the emotional comfort and sense of fulfillment that come from warm human contact, creative expression, and spiritual connection. We will, more than likely, eat in an unhealthy way if we do not nourish ourselves on other levels.

Those Elusive Instincts

Since I consider our instincts to be important to healthy eating, I devoted all of chapter 11 to this subject. Why did we lose access to our food instinct? One obvious reason is the loss of our ancestral food. The other reason is that our emotional needs have become entangled with our nutritional needs. In fact, I have suggested that emotional unrest might be the single most important factor that makes healthy eating difficult. This is a major reason that "diets don't work." As we make peace with ourselves, our chosen diet probably *will* work, because our instincts can finally kick in, and guide us to fulfill our true nutritional needs.

In other words, to fulfill our nutritional needs, we also have to give proper attention to our true emotional needs. Ultimately, our emotional needs have to do with relationship — with each other and the rest of Life. The latter has to do the humane and environmental considerations discussed in the previous chapter.

The Outer Reflects the Inner

One of the points made in the previous chapter is that the same food choices that promote the life within us, also blesses the life around us. What's good for you is good for your neighbor. What is good for you and your neighbor is good for the Earth and the living beings upon it.

I have written this book because I, like so many others, have often found it challenging to consistently eat in ways that promote optimum health. Why is it so hard? Why is it not as natural for humans to eat healthfully? Why does it often prove to be as futile as pulling ourselves up by our own boot straps? The answer: We find it challenging to eat healthfully for essentially the same reason we are inclined to ignore or forget the ethical considerations of eating. In other words, the same mechanism that causes us to forget how to eat for health also causes us to forget how to be good stewards of the land and good neighbors to each other. We can sum it up with one word — addiction.

We are trying to solve our health and social problems with a mind that is addicted to the very same substances and conditions that cause or aggravate the problems. It's like putting a liquor manufacturer in charge of Alcoholics Anonymous.

In the Belly of the Beast

It is exceedingly difficult to consistently eat healthfully when we are addicted to foods and other substances that hurt the body. Likewise, our attempts to create peace, social justice, and sustainable methods of food production have apparently been futile because we have been trying to do so with political institutions and economic systems that are addicted to war, exploitation and overconsumption.

To complicate matters, personal and social addictions do not merely parallel each other; they are very much intertwined. The same addictions that stimulate or sedate our senses also result in the numbing of our natural sensibilities, loss of conscience, and clouding of our power of discernment. Therefore, we blindly abuse our bodies, each other, and the environment that supports us.

With addiction comes a growing lethargy and misting of the mind. When addiction is deep enough, we become oblivious to the consequences our actions. The only thing that seems to matter is immediate gratification.

If we try to fight back, we discover that resistance is worse than futile, because the more we fight the addiction, the stronger it seems to get, apparently thriving on our efforts to overcome it. For example, addiction seems to feed on the very guilt we often feel when we "slip."

As our energy becomes depleted, and power of discernment wanes, we experience an increasing indifference, or flat-out denial, of how our actions undermine our personal health, hurt others, and damage the very environment that sustains us.

Addiction enslaves all of us — including those who appear to be the enslavers, for they too are addicted. Addiction locks us into a state of immaturity and helplessness, slowing down our natural progression from childhood to the creative passion of the responsible adult, and eventually into the wisdom and deep tranquility of the elder.

For all these reasons, any addiction, whether it is personal or societal, should be approached with patience, thoughtfulness, and care. "Cold turkey" is not necessarily a good idea. The longer we are addicted to anything, the trickier it is to untangle ourselves from it. Freeing ourselves from an addition is a bit like getting off a moving merry-go-round — one that spins faster, the longer we stay on it!

Addictions to wheat, meat, and war have been with us a very long time. They form a three-tiered merry-go-round that has been spinning ever faster for an estimated 10,000 years, and possibly longer. That same merry-go-round has also been propelled by other addictive substances that have been added over the centuries — refined sugar, alcohol, tobacco, caffeine, opium, etc. Such substances have been the basis for much of the conquest, slavery, and other forms of exploitation, throughout history.

The merry-go-round is like a great beast that holds us in its belly, and continuously draws power from us. On the social level, the beast is a global economy that is addicted to war and ever-increasing consumption, which, in turn, are driven by our everyday personal addictions.

To Fight the Beast is to Feed the Beast

How do we stop feeding a beast whose appetite controls our capacity to experience pleasure and pain? How do we fight it, when it seems to feed on the attacks leveled against it? Below is a quote from a well-known historical figure who tried gallantly to fight the beast on the societal level, and inspired many others to do the same.

"I am as desirous of being a good neighbor as I am of being a bad subject."
— Henry David Thoreau

In one sense, Mr. Thoreau was the archetypal image of American idealism — free thinking, pioneering, self-responsible, idealistic and intensely moral. He was a role model of the good citizen and thoughtful neighbor. He was an extraordinary example of one individual who tread to think globally and act locally. His solution was to dare to challenge the all too common personal and societal addictions that destroy our personal health, pollute the planet, and undermine social justice.

Mr. Thoreau fine-tuned and integrated his ideas during his two-year stay at Walden Pond, in the 1840s. During that time period, he built his own house and grew most of his own food. He was blessed with an abundance of solitude to clear his mind. His diet was simpler, cleaner, and more nutritious than that of his fellow citizens. He generally abstained from alcohol, tobacco, coffee, and other stimulants and depressants that were regularly used by others. He had effectively distanced himself from the addictions to the various conveniences and forms of pacification of the day — many of which were dependent on slavery and other forms of exploitation.

During his extended retreat at Walden Pond, his perspective on life deepened and moved further away from the beaten path. Not surprisingly, after Mr. Thoreau left Walden, he eventually found himself in jail. What did he do? He refused to pay a certain tax, which he felt supported slavery — a vice that he fiercely attacked, because it so blatantly contradicted the founding principles of the United States, which he deeply respected.

While in jail, he was visited by another giant of American literature, Ralph Waldo Emerson. Mr. Emerson exclaimed, "Henry, what are you doing in there?" The prisoner responded, "Waldo, what are *you* doing out *there*?"

Henry David Thoreau's efforts were noble. His insights are priceless. He quietly influenced many social activists in the years that followed, well into the 20th century, and even to the present time. However, his impact, like that of other reformers and advocates of social justice, was limited by his very efforts to fight the beast.

Here Is the Good News

The simple answer to the paradox described above is that we automatically stop feeding the beast, when we start nourishing our spirit. Reclaiming our spiritual life can begin to un-dam our emotional waters, so they flow naturally in the direction of unity, thus allowing us to evolve in the direction of Henry David Thoreau's vision of the ideal citizen — free thinking, self-responsible, and ever respectful of one's neighbor.

Those who are seriously committed to 12-step programs are keenly aware that reclaiming one's spiritual life is essential to recovery. I am of the opinion that personal health, as well as our relationships with each other and the planet, are all nicely addressed and integrated when enough humans answer their personal inner call to awaken spiritually.

As I have previously suggested, a healthy spiritual life is the key to healthy eating, because without it, emotional energy is effectively dammed — it cannot flow to its natural destination. The mind becomes waterlogged with troubled emotions and unfulfilled desires, which obscure our thinking, break our will, and drown our eating instincts.

As described in chapter 11, spiritual awakening simply means that your emotional energy is allowed to flow freely, and return home. Spiritual awakening does not have to be formalized. Neither does it have to be heavy or gloomy. Neither does it even have to be called "spiritual." It is often experienced as a simple calming of the mind and awakening of the heart. We might experience it as a softening of our gaze and easing of our harsh demands on ourselves and others. We simply "lighten up."

In its most pristine form, spiritual awakening might show up as a simple feeling that seems to emerge from nowhere; an innocent and perhaps childlike sense of being warmly connected to the people, animals, and even plants around us. On a more subtle level, it might show up as a more detached, non-personal, and perhaps agnostic set of values that preclude the possibility of mistreating the life around us. Or, it can be based on a deeply personal belief in the God of our understanding.

In other words, regardless of the form it takes, spiritual connection, expressed in practical terms, shows up as a more honest and respectful relationship with everything and everyone. Relationship of any kind is about being responsible. With a return of our sense spiritual connection comes an awakening of our true responsibility to our own bodies and the life around us — including the people who bring food to us. With such awakening, we do not have to make ourselves act responsibly, for it is as natural to us as eating when we are hungry, and drinking when we are thirsty.

Our Origins and Destiny

Spiritual cultivation provides the stabilizing and unifying force that integrates all the other elements of life, including our relationship to food, and to each other. With such a foundation in place, spiritual cultivation naturally evolves, and eventually expresses as a deep hunger to discover our origins and fulfill our destiny.

This might seem like a lofty pursuit, far removed from the practical matters of everyday life, however, if we do not answer that inner call, everything we do to maintain health will break down, including our choice to eat healthy. The body cannot be well nourished if the soul is starved. If that inner hunger is neglected or suppressed, we become self-destructive, individually and collectively.

Spiritual awakening eventually compels us to recognize our past, and make peace with it. None of it is cast out. We realize that every bit of it contributes to our lives. All of it is transformed into the fertile soil of our personal and cultural landscape, which makes our human existence rich and meaningful.

To fulfill our destiny, we must remember our roots — simply because our destiny will ultimately resemble our roots. Looking at it from a broader perspective, evolution seems to occur in spirals, wherein the patterns of the past reemerge later on higher levels. We can see this in the overall evolution of life on Earth.[1]

In light of this, I find it interesting that more and more humans are rediscovering the virtues of unprocessed fruits and vegetables, whether it is for reasons of personal health, ecological sustainability, humane concerns, or spiritual cultivation. The ecological garden seems to be a common gathering point for all these needs. Also, from a purely aesthetic standpoint, there is a certain poetic appeal to the elegance and symmetry of "returning to the garden" to receive our food, as well as the inspiration and guidance to proceed on our collective evolutionary journey.

As suggested in Chapter 7, our human origins, as described by the theory of evolution, have some intriguing similarities to the account given in the Biblical story of Genesis. Both point to fruits and vegetables as being our original foods. Chapter 7 also describes how primates evolved to be in relationship with fruit trees — a relationship that became so deep and intimate over an estimated 65 million years, that it can be called symbiotic. Primates and fruit trees evolved together and apparently drove each other's evolution. Primates helped shape the tropical forests of today; just as fruit trees shaped the evolution of the primate body and behavior. Primates cannot help but be good stewards of the forest, because they are biologically designed for the job.

We are primates. It would be contrary to the evidence before us to deny or disown our relationship with the natural world, especially the forest. Granted, our sense of connection might be so deeply buried in our psyche as to make us oblivious to it, but it is still fundamental to our nature. It is encoded in our DNA, written in our bones, and flows through our blood. We see evidence of it in our declining health through eating processed foods. We see it as a loss of sanity, a sense of vague anxiety, restlessness, and alienation when we spend too much time in artificial environments — we feel like strangers in a strange land of our own making. The lack of ease might be exceedingly subtle and easy to ignore. As we plod on through our concrete jungles, the feeling might be beyond our capacity to describe in words, but if it could speak, it might say, "I feel lost here. I want to go home."

We also see it in the restoration of health through eating fresh whole foods straight from the garden. We experience it as a clearing of the mind and a softening of the emotions when we reconnect with the natural world. This might be why we instinctively seek relatively undeveloped and richly foliated settings to promote a calming of the mind, and to facilitate spiritual remembrance. Monasteries and retreats are often established in pristine environments. It is not merely for the sake of solitude. The inner call to mature spiritually is about relaxing our outer striving and returning home to our true nature — which seems to occur most easily when we connect *with* Nature.

This brings us back to permaculture, described in the previous chapter. Permaculture encourages us to relax and observe Nature, so we can learn to cooperate with it. With permaculture, we have a practical way to enjoy the bounties that Nature is ever ready to bestow on us, rather than settling for crumbs stolen from our neighbor's table.

Childhood's End

On the scientific level, permaculture reminds us of ecological succession, from bare ground to grassland, to scrubland, and finally to the maturity and stability of the forest. This natural maturation of the land is restricted only by lack of water and sun — or humans fastidiously holding it back through great effort and expense — insisting that the land remain "immature" as a pasture, a wheat field, or a perfectly manicured but otherwise useless lawn. Such treatment of the land might serve to remind us of how we often expend a lot of energy, and ultimately hold back our own spiritual maturation, for the sake of appearance and short-term material gain. In fact, as many individuals eventually discover, our relentless drive for material gain, sometimes turns our inner terrain into a spiritual wasteland, just as our collective drive for conquest and wealth have historically turned fertile land into desert.

The rebirth of permaculture principles may be metaphorically seen as a sort of "maturing" of the synergistic relationship that has existed between fruit trees and our ancestors for tens of millions years. For humans, being good stewards of Earth is a logical extension of the natural role of primates in the wild. With humans, that same capacity may be said to have awakened — or is trying to. What other primates do instinctively, we can do intentionally, and in a way that is unique to our humanity.

What will we do when we are able to stop our spiritual wandering through the desert of our own making, and finally return to our home in the Garden? What will we do with the newly rediscovered sense of peace and power that come from being as intimately connected to our spiritual identity as we are to the Earth that feeds us? I don't know. However, to paraphrase Arthur C. Clark, I suspect we will think of something.[2]

Appendix A
Food Combining For Digestion Perfection
by David Klein, Ph.D.

    Food combining is the consumption of foods that are compatible with our digestive physiology. While mono meals (one type of food per meal) yield the best results, simple meals of 2 or 3 different compatible foods also work well. We cannot completely digest complex food combinations, as evidenced by indigestion, acid reflux, diarrhea, body odors, flu, pimples, fatigue, etc. This is because meals of improperly combined foods limit digestion — the foods decompose (rot) in the gut, poisoning us and potentially leading to irritable bowel, colitis, Crohn's disease, GERD, and many other gastrointestinal diseases. In fact, Hygienic physiologists agree that over ninety percent of all known common maladies and major diseases are caused by autointoxication, i.e., self-poisoning, mainly from eating diets that are incompatible with our constitutions. The old Chinese saying holds true: "Disease enters through the mouth."

    Starch digestion begins in the mouth. We must chew starchy food well, mix it with saliva. Our salivary enzymes are alkaline, and are weakened when mixed with acids. Therefore, we must not consume acid fruits with starchy foods.

    Hydrochloric acid and an enzyme, called pepsin, are secreted in the stomach when we eat high-protein foods (e.g., nuts, seeds, and avocados). If we eat starchy foods with high-protein foods, the alkaline salivary enzymes will mix with the acidic stomach enzymes in the stomach, curtailing digestion, causing the starches to ferment and proteins to putrefy in the gut. Thus, it is obvious that nuts and white potatoes or grains cannot digest well together. This also applies to the conventional combinations of meat with potatoes, pasta with meatballs, pizza with cheese and meat, hamburgers and hot dogs on buns, meat and bread sandwiches with mayonnaise, cereal with milk, and rice with tofu or beans.

    Fruits are essentially predigested, requiring little digestive effort. Their nutrients need to be absorbed into the bloodstream within 10 to 60 minutes;

otherwise they ferment. The denser, bulkier fruits that have a bit of fat, such as bananas, require the longest retention time in the stomach (about an hour), where they are mixed with a small amount of water and gradually released into the small intestine. Fruits digest best by themselves or with green vegetables (celery, lettuce, and kale), because their starch, protein, and fat content is low and, thus, their digestion will not interfere with the digestion of fruit. In fact, the inclusion of greens with fruit meals generally aids digestion by virtue of their fiber and complementary nutrient content.

The fat in fatty foods (most of which are also high in protein) is primarily digested in the upper part of the small intestine. When large complex meals are eaten, the food will be held up in the stomach for many hours and the fat will likely become rancid and rendered unusable before it can be digested. The complete digestion of starch, protein, and fat requires time — approximately 1 to 2 hours for raw food meals and several hours longer for cooked foods. The digestion of these nutrients also requires full-strength enzymatic action. If starchy and fatty high-protein foods are ingested with water, beverages, and watery fruit, the additional liquid content will dilute the concentration of the digestive enzymes, reducing their effectiveness.

If sweet, non-acid fruit is eaten with large portions of starchy and/or fatty high-protein foods, they will be detained for more than an hour in the stomach and will transit more slowly through the bowel. Their sugars will ferment, potentially causing all sorts of problems, including irritable bowel, yeast overgrowth, gassiness, diarrhea, vomiting, and brain fog. Furthermore, simultaneous high concentrations of sugar and fat in the bloodstream causes problems with blood sugar metabolism, such as diabetes.

If small portions of starchy and/or fatty high-protein foods are eaten with large portions of sweet fruits or juices, this hinders the body's ability to sense the presence of the starch, protein, and fat. The digestive enzymes they require may not be secreted, and fermentation and putrefaction will likely occur. As an example, nuts/seeds/butters/avocado added to sweet, non-acid fruit smoothies will not be digested. The combining of minimal amounts of acid fruits with fatty-protein foods (such as in a salad dressing) tends to digest well for some people because the acids in the fruits aid in the breaking down of protein molecules.

David Klein is the author of "Self Healing Colitis & Crohn's" and "Digestion Perfection."
To read Dr. Klein's full article on food combining and get the laminated version of his food combining chart, please visit http://www.colitis-crohns.com.

Appendix B
The Enzymes in Raw Foods

Enzymes are protein molecules that promote the chemicals reactions that make life possible. All living animals, plants and microbes produce enzymes. Some enzymes are used to digest food, while other are used to power other important metabolic processes, such as destroying cancer cells, getting rid of infections, and promoting regeneration.

Enzymes molecules tend to be very delicate, and are destroyed when heated too far beyond normal physiological temperatures. Normal cooking destroys all enzymes. Not surprisingly, some raw food enthusiasts promote the benefits of enzymes in raw foods. Critics respond by saying that such enzymes are for the use of the plant only, and are destroyed by the acids in the stomach. Yes, many of enzymes in raw foods are for plant use only, such as the ones that promote the ripening of fruit. However, raw plant food also contains digestive enzymes that apparently do remain functional when we eat them.

Plant digestive enzymes are functional in the upper portion of the stomach, where food may be processed for about an hour. The enzymes then become non-functional in the lower acidic portion of the stomach, and become active again in the small intestine, to help with further digestion. They can also be absorbed into the blood stream, where they remain functional, and are used by the body. For example, pineapples contain a protein-digesting enzyme, called bromelain, which helps to digest protein, as well as reducing painful inflammation in joints and other injured tissues.

Appendix C

Sour Power
by Lupa Idri

For ages, humans have used fermented foods to improve intestinal health, as these foods help replenish the friendly bacteria in our digestive tracts. Many cultures worldwide consider fermented foods a normal part of life. In Russia, a fermented combination of vegetables is their national dish, and cultured veggies are served with every meal throughout the Baltic regions of Eastern Europe. In fact, the people of Bulgarian and Asian descent are known for their longevity, which many attribute to their consumption of fermented foods.

Benefits of fermented vegetables
- Foods that undergo fermentation are easier to digest and more nutritious.
- Fermentation improves the bioavailability of minerals present in our food.
- Fermentation creates new nutrients and other beneficial substances, such as omega-3 fats, SOD, glutathione, phospholipids, digestive enzymes, and beta 2.3 glucans.
- Ferments, such as cultured beets or gingered carrots, are sources of antioxidants, which scavenge cancer precursors, known as free radicals, from the cell of the body.
- The sour taste of fermented foods is due to the production of lactic acid by bacteria. Lactic acid promotes intestinal motility, as well as discourages the growth of harmful intestinal organisms associated with diarrhea, such as Shigella, Salmonella, and E. coli.

How to Make Sauerkraut
- One 2 lb. cabbage head — shredded
- Himalayan salt —1 Tbs. per 2 lb. of cabbage
- 2 teaspoons caraway seed — optional
- Mix ingredients in large bowl and add 4 Tbs. whey

- Pound cabbage from 7-10 minutes to bruise the cabbage and get the juices running, which is needed for proper fermentation
- Pack in Mason jars. Keep the lids loose, so the fermenting veggies can "breath."
- Store at 68-72 degrees for 3 days, then refrigerate for a week or longer.
- Using the same basic process described above, you can ferment any vegetable or combinations of vegetables, such cauliflower, beets, carrots, and cucumbers.

Appendix D
Food and Cardiovascular Health

Since cardiovascular disease is currently the number one cause of death in industrialized societies, and since the food connection has some controversy and confusion, this subject merits close examination.

The Confusion
Here is the potentially confusing part of cardiovascular health: On the one hand, traditional diets throughout the world that are low in saturated fats and cholesterol are associated with longevity and decreased risk of cardiovascular disease.[4] These finding have been substantiated by controlled studies in industrialized nations.[5] Likewise, diets that are high in saturated fats and cholesterol show greater overall mortality rate and increased risk of cardiovascular disease.[6] On the other hand, high levels of saturated fats and cholesterol are not the primary cause of arterial plaquing, and the overall effects of cholesterol-lowering drugs in preventing heart attacks has been dismal.

The answer to this puzzle is actually quite simple. The fact that diets high in saturated fat and cholesterol are associated with higher incidents of cardiovascular disease does not necessarily mean that these fats actually *cause* the condition. In other words, the high cholesterol level is a useful marker for *predicting* cardiovascular disease, which is different from saying that it is an actual cause. There might be other factors riding along with the fats that actually trigger the condition. If that is the case, taking drugs to lower the blood lipids, while doing nothing else, is sheer folly. Which brings us to the controversy...

The Controversy
Starting in the 1960s, the primary emphasis in the prevention of heart disease has been the managing of blood cholesterol levels through the use of drugs. However, after decades of relying on such treatment, the weight of the evidence

seems to be shouting at us to change our ways. Fifty years of relying on such therapy has produced very poor results.

Firstly, the evidence suggests that cholesterol and saturated fats are not the primary causes of cardiovascular disease. In fact, one study found that older individuals with lower cholesterol levels had a *greater* risk of death than those with higher cholesterol.[1]

In light of all this, the use of cholesterol lowering drugs as the primary preventive treatment for cardiovascular disease defies common sense. No major study has proven that statins lowers the risk of dying from any condition, except perhaps in males who have already suffered one or more heart attacks.[2] Some studies even suggest that lowering the cholesterol through certain drugs actually *increases* arterial plaquing.[3] Furthermore, cholesterol lowering drugs (statins) have a number of side effects:

- Memory loss
- Type 2 diabetes
- Sore muscles
- Fatigue
- Lack of endurance
- Reduced capacity to store glycogen in the muscles
- Working out while on statins is more difficult, and post-workout muscle recovery takes a longer time. This is significant when we remember that exercise promotes the balancing of blood lipids.

When we factor in the side effects of these drugs, we are faced with the possibility that, overall, they have done more harm than good. In addition to the actual harm done by the drugs, the individual seeking help for cardiovascular disease is being diverted from the real causes and real solutions, described below.

The Causes of Cardiovascular Disease

Inflammation is the key. The primary factor that triggers the formation of plaque in arteries is the irritation and subsequent inflammation of their inner lining.[7] Once the inflammation is established, it tends to perpetuate itself, leading to the growth of arterial plaques, consisting of mostly of fibrotic material and fat, including a goodly amount of cholesterol.

Here are the specific dietary factors that contribute to the chronic low-grade inflammation and subsequent plaquing of arteries.

- **Lack of vitamin C** and related phytonutrients. Vitamin C and associated flavonoids are essential for the production of collagen, which is a major building material for blood vessels.[8]

- **Lack of omega-3 oils.** These important oils keep inflammation in check and help maintain the smoothness and elasticity of the inner lining of blood vessels.[9]
- **Lack of dietary antioxidants.** Much of the damage that leads to inflammation and plaquing is caused or accelerated by free-radical damage.[10]
- **Lack of vitamin B12 and folate** can lead to high levels of homocysteine, which is a major irritant for the inner lining of blood vessels.
- **Too many pro-inflammatory foods and not enough anti-inflammatory foods.** In other words, too much dairy, grains, refined vegetable oils high in omega-6 (safflower and corn oil), animal protein, and not enough fruits and vegetables. Stated differently, too much of the macronutrients and not enough micronutrients.

High Levels of Saturated Fats and Cholesterol Are Okay?

To properly address this question, we have to be willing to consider the possibility that the answer is not going to be as simple as "yes" or "no." Also, for those who have looked into this deeply enough to have an opinion, it is important that we free ourselves of the notion that we already know the answer.

Firstly, opinions vary as to what constitutes a "healthy level." To further complicate matters, the question of individual differences is typically ignored. Also, though high levels of these fats may not be the primary cause of arterial plaquing, they might contribute to it directly or indirectly:

- Even if the fats themselves are totally benign at high levels, the same diet that is loaded with these fats is likely to have other factors that can contribute to cardiovascular disease, such as sodium, oxidized cholesterol, and heme iron.
- The typical diet high in saturated fat and cholesterol also tends to be high in sodium, which stiffens the arteries and contributes to high blood pressure, both of which can irritate and injure the inner lining of arteries.
- High levels of cholesterol (even if harmless, in and of itself) are likely to expose the body to more *oxidized* cholesterol, which has been shown to trigger arterial plaquing.[11] Animal studies suggest that a relatively small amount of oxidized cholesterol (0.3% of ingested cholesterol) can cause damage to the walls of arteries.[12] Cholesterol is oxidized by cooking, especially at high temperatures, as in broiling, deep-frying, and industrial canning.

- High levels of heme iron (found in red meat) can trigger oxidation of cholesterol.[13]
- Some studies suggest that high levels of saturated and monounsaturated fats impede the dilation of arteries.[14]
- High levels of saturated fats and cholesterol have a tendency to thicken the blood, which, in turn, tends to increase blood pressure, raise the risk of clot formation, and stress the delicate inner lining of the blood vessels.
- High levels of dietary saturated fats and cholesterol are associated with insulin resistance, which results in chronically high insulin levels. Some studies suggest that a meal dominated by animal products can raise insulin even more than a plate of pasta.[15] Chronically high insulin levels can compromise the integrity of the inner lining of blood vessels.

The Good News

Though the mechanisms that contribute to arterial plaquing are more complex than once believed, the solution is still very simple, and may be summarized with a single word: FOOD. Making the proper dietary adjustments has been shown to be effective in preventing and reversing cardiovascular disease, especially when supported by exercise and stress reduction techniques, such as meditation and yoga.

Overall, the low-fat, plant-based diets have yielded the most consistent results in reversing cardiovascular disease. However, low-carb (high-fat) diets have also been used successfully.[15] Either way, the key is to make sure the carbs and fats are of the healthy whole-food variety, while being moderate with protein and animal products, and making room for generous helpings of fresh fruits and vegetables, especially the latter.

Endnotes and References

Chapter 3

1. Bazzano LA, Li TY, Joshipura KJ, et al. Intake of Fruit, Vegetables, and Fruit Juices and *Risk of Diabetes in Women. Diabetes Care* 2008; 31: 1311–1317.
2. Hancock CR, Han DH, Chen M, Terada S, Yasuda T, Wright DC, Holloszy JO. High-fat diets cause insulin resistance despite an increase in muscle mitochondria. *Proc Natl Acad Sci..* 2008. Jun 3; 105(22): 7815–20.
3. Blaylock, Russell L. *Health and Nutrition Secrets that can Save Your Life.* Albuquerque, NM. Health Press, 2006. Pp 293–294.
4. Vogel, Robert, A. Brachial Artery Ultrasound: A Noninvasive Tool in Assessment of Triglyceride Rich Lipoproteins. *Clinical Cardiology.* June 1999.
5. Brown BG, Taylor AJ, Does ENHANCE Diminish Confidence in Lowering LDL or in Ezetimibe? Engl J Med 358:1504, April 3, 2008 Editorial.
6. Abramson J, Wright JM. Are lipid-lowering guidelines evidence-based? *Lancet.* 2007 Jan 20; 369(9557): 168–9.
7. Esselstyn, Caldwell, B. *Prevent and Reverse Heart Disease.* 31–32. Every Books. New York. 2007. p 75.
8. Cannon, Christopher P., et al. Intensive vs Moderate Lipid Lowering with Statins After Acute Coronary Syndrome. *New England Journal of Medicine.* 4/8/2004.
9. Are trans-fatty acids a serious risk for disease? Discussion. Am J Clin Nutr 1997 66:18S–1019S.
10. AIlona Staprans; Xian-Mang Pan; Joseph H. Rapp; Kenneth R. Feingold. Oxidized. Cholesterol in the Diet Accelerates the

Development of Aortic Atherosclerosis in Cholesterol-Fed Rabbits. *Arteriosclerosis, Thrombosis, and Vascular Biology.* 1998; 18: 977–983.).
11. Siddons, RC. Et al. The experimental production of vitamin B_{12} deficiency in the baboon. A 2-year study. *Br J Nutr.* 1974 Sep; 32 (2): 219–28.
12. Milton, K (2003). "Micronutrient intakes of wild primates: are humans different? *Comparative Biochemistry and Physiology.* 136 (1): 47–59.
13. Levine M, Dhariwal KR, Washko PW, Butler JD, Welch RW, WangYH, Bergsten P. Ascorbic acid and in situ kinetics: a new approach to vitamin requirements. *Am J Clin Nutr* December 1991 54: 1157S–1162S.

Chapter 4

1. GMO corn has been altered to produce a toxin that makes holes in the digestive systems of bugs that attack corn plants. This toxin allegedly also attacks human intestines, and has recently been shown to have the capacity to modify the DNA of human intestinal bacteria, so that your own normal bacteria thereafter continually poisons you. These claims are challenged by the producers of GMO foods.
2. Spiroux, J. Roullier, F. Cellier, D., Séralini, G. E. A Comparison of the Effects of Three GM Corn Varieties on Mammalian Health. *Int J Biol Sci* 2009; 5(7): 706–726. doi:10.7150/ijbs.5.706.
3. Arshi, M., Afaq, F., Sarfaraz, S., Adhami, V.M., Syed, D.N. Mukhtar, H. Pomegranate fruit juice for chemoprevention and chemotherapy of prostate cancer. *PNAS* 2005 102 (41) 14813–14818.
4. The Dangers of Raw Milk: Unpasteurized Milk Can Pose a Serious Health Risk. (From FDA website)
5. Siegal-Itzkovich. J. Health committee warns of potential dangers of soya. *BMJ* 2005; 331 doi: http://dx.doi.org/10.1136/bmj.331.7511.254-a (Published 28 July 2005)

Chapter 5

1. Bernard, N. *Reversing Type II Diabetes.* Pp 22–23. Rodale Press 2007.
2. Peterson, K. F, et al. Impaired Mitochondrial Activity in the Insulin-Resistant Offspring of Patients with Type II Diabetes. *New England Journal of Medicine* 350 (2004): 664–71.

3. Wolpert HA, et al. Dietary Fat Acutely Increases Glucose Concentrations and Insulin Requirements in Patients with Type I Diabetes: Implications for carbohydrate-based bolus dose calculation and intensive diabetes management. *Diabetes Care.* 2012 Nov 27. [Epub ahead of print]. Joslin Diabetes Center, Boston, Massachusetts.
4. Martinez-Outschoorn UE, Lin Z, Whitaker-Menezes D, Howell A, Sotgia F, Lisanti MP. Ketone body utilization drives tumor growth and metastasis. *Cell Cycle.* 2012 Sep 19; 11(21).
5. Parrett, Owens, S. Why I Am a Vegetarian. From essay published on website.
6. Kouchakoff M.D. The Influence of Food Cooking on the Blood Formula of Man. Institute of Clinical Chemistry, Lausanne, Switzerland, Proceedings: First International Congress of Microbiology, Paris 1930. "After every dose of food, we also observe a general augmentation of white corpuscles, and a change in the correlation of their percentage. This phenomenon has been considered, until now, a physiological one, and is called a digestive leukocytosis. After the consumption of the same natural foodstuffs, altered by means of high temperature, we find that the general number of white corpuscles has changed, but the correlation of their percentage has remained the same. After consumption of manufactured foodstuffs not only has the number of white corpuscles changed but also the correlation of percentage between them. All our experiments have shown that it is not the quantity, but the quality of food which plays an important role in the alteration of our blood formula, and that 200 milligrams or even 50 milligrams of foodstuffs produce the same reaction as large doses of them."
7. Pottenger, F.M. *"Pottenger's Cats: A Study in Nutrition."* This is a summary of Dr. Pottenger's 10-year, multigenerational nutrition study on cats, compiled by the Price-Pottenger Nutrition Foundation. 1983.
8. Mucc, LA, Dickman, PW, Steineck, G, Adami H-O, Augustsson, K. Dietary acrylamide and cancer of the large bowel, kidney, and bladder: Absence of an association in a population-based study in Sweden. *British Journal of Cancer* (2003) 88, 84–89. doi:10.1038/sj.bjc.6600726.
9. Sherwin, E.R. Oxidation and antioxidants in fat and oil processing. *Journal of the American Oil Chemists' Society.* Volume 55, Number 11 (1978), 809–814, DOI: 10.1007/BF02682653.

10. Koschinsky, T, He, CJ, Mitsuhashi, T, Bucala, R, Liu, C, Buenting C, Heitmann K, Vlassara H (1997). Orally absorbed reactive glycation products (glycotoxins): an environmental risk factor in diabetic nephropathy. *Proceedings of the National Academy of Sciences* 94 (12): 6474–9. doi:10.1073/pnas.94.12.6474. PMC 21074. PMID 9177242.

Chapter 6

1. John P. Reganold, Preston K. Andrews, Jennifer R. Reeve, Lynne Carpenter-Boggs, Christopher W. Schadt, J. Richard Alldredge, Carolyn F. Ross, Neal M. Davies, and Jizhong Zhou, . Fruit and Soil Quality of Organic and Conventional Strawberry Agroecosystems. *Plos ONE*, September 2010, Vol. 5, Issue 9.
2. Sherman, JD. 1996 Chlorpyrifos (Dursban)-associated birth defects: report of four cases. *Arch. Env. Health* 51(1): 5–8).

Chapter 7

1. Rafert, J. Vineberg, E.O. Bonobo Nutrition — relation of captive diet to wild diet. *Bonobo Husbandry Manual*, American Association of Zoos and Aquariums. 1997.
2. The anthropoids were already pre-adapted for life on the ground. Their grasping hands and nimble fingers were perfect for plucking edible shrubs, and picking berries and mushrooms. Their stereoscopic color vision, which served them well in the trees, was also useful on the ground for spotting predators — and to allow some Hominids to eventually become hunters themselves. Furthermore, the same muscles used for swinging through the branches, were also perfectly suited for swinging a club.
3. Koops. K, McGrew. W , Matsuzawa. T, Knapp. L, *Terrestrial Nest-Building by Wild Chimpanzees (Pan troglodytes): Implications for the Tree-to-Ground Sleep Transition in Early Hominins*, American Journal of Physical Anthropology. April 2012, DOI: 10.1002/ajpa.22056.
4. Even when the fruit trees were fairly plentiful, our ancestors may have grown to a size that made it easier to climb down to the ground to forage berries and low-hanging branches, or walk to the next tree.[5] In other words, greater body-size, with a disproportionally large brain

was simply the way primates had been evolving for millions of years, long before the forests began thinning out. Larger size would have given them an advantage over competing fruit eaters and other threats, as well as making them even more efficient at spreading the seeds of their preferred fruit trees.

5. Origins of Human Bipedalism. Nova. (From Website).
6. Sponheimer, M., Lee-Thorp, J. A. Isotopic Evidence for the Diet of an Early Hominid, Australopithecus africanus. *Science* 15 January 1999: Vol. 283 no. 5400 pp. 368–370.
7. Milton, K. Hunter-gatherer diets; a different perspective. *American Journal of Clinic Nutrition* 2000. 71:665.
8. Stahl, A.B. Hominid Dietary Selection Before Fire. *Current Anthropology.* Vol 5 #2. April 1984.
9. Milton, K. Diversity of plant foods in tropical forests as a stimulus to mental development in primates. *American Anthropologist* 1981; 83(3): 534–548.
10. Gorman, R. M. "Cooking up Bigger Brains." *Scientific American,* December 2007.
11. Henry AG, Brooks AS, Piperno DR. Microfossils in calculus demonstrate consumption of plants and cooked foods in Neanderthal diets. *National Academy of Science.* 2011 Jan 11; 108(2):486–91.
12. Ilona Staprans; Xian-Mang Pan; Joseph H. Rapp; Kenneth R. Feingold. Oxidized. Cholesterol in the Diet Accelerates the Development of Aortic Atherosclerosis in Cholesterol-Fed Rabbits. *Arteriosclerosis, Thrombosis, and Vascular Biology.* 1998; 18: 977–983.)
13. Mercader J. Mozambican grass seed consumption during the Middle Stone Age. *Science.* 2009 Dec 18; 326(5960):1680–3.
14. Tang, G. Bioconversion of dietary provitamin A carotenoids to vitamin A in Humans. *American Journal of Clinical Nutrition* 2010; 91(suppl):1468S–73S.
15. The alleged degeneration includes an actual shrinking of the brain. Looking at figure 7, the short horizontal line (indicating the stoppage of brain growth in the last 200,000 years) should actually be going down!
16. Berry R. *Food for the Gods: Vegetarianism & the World's Religions.* Pythagorean Publishers. 1998

17. Wright, A, Gynn, G. *Left in the Dark*. Kaleodis Press, 2008. Chapter 3. According to the primary author, Tony Wright, we became fully human in the forest, not in the savanna! This is radically different from mainstream paleontology. He suggests that the prime real estate (food-wise) would have been in the forest, therefore, that is where the biggest, strongest, and smartest hominids would have lived. He also suggests that the fossils that were found in the savannas of old were those of less well-adapted hominids that were forced to leave the forest — and eventually became extinct. He also says that we have not found human remains in the forest for the same reason that we have not found chimp and gorilla fossils — the bones decompose too easily.
18. Wright, A, Gynn, G. *Left in the Dark*. Kaleodis Press, 2008. Pg 189. The author points out that the extremely rapid brain growth in early humans is consistent with the exponential growth seen in any positive feedback loop, well known to physiologists. Any positive feedback loop eventually results in exponential growth, if allowed to continue in an unrestricted manner. In this case, the author asserts that the millions of years of eating tropical fruits and vegetables by our primate ancestors set up a positive feedback loop. The steady diet of fruit and other tropical plant foods influenced hormonal levels, which in turn influenced gene expression in such a way as to allow for greater development of the brain and pineal gland. This further influenced hormonal levels and gene expression, which allowed for and even bigger brain and pineal gland, etc. This positive feedback loop supposedly occurred faster and faster over tens of millions of years of primate evolution, resulting in rapid brain growth, until finally the growth became exponential, resulting in the huge brain of humans.
19. Wright, A, Gynn, G. *Left in the Dark*. Kaleodis Press, 2008. Pp 75–77.
20. Lipton, B.H., Bhaerman, S. *Spontaneous Evolution*. Hay House. 2009. Pp 132–142. Since epigenetic adaptations can be passed on to the next generation, it can theoretically allow a species to evolve much faster than allowed by Darwinian evolution, and therefore, possibly explain the exponential brain growth in early humans.
21. From the Weston A. Price Foundation Website.
22. Milton, K., Nutritional Characteristics of Wild Primate Foods: Do the Diets of Our Closest Living Relatives Have Lessons for Us? *Nutrition* 1999; 15: 488–498. ©Elsevier Science Inc. 1999

Chapter 8

1. From *The 80/10/10 Diet*, by Dr. Douglass Graham. Pg 27.

Chapter 9

1. Lagiou, P., Sandin, S., et al. Low carbohydrate-high protein diet and incidence of cardiovascular diseases in Swedish women: prospective cohort study. *BMJ 2012; 344.*
2. Fung T.T, van Dam R.M., Hankinson S.E, et al. Low-Carbohydrate Diets and All-Cause and Cause-Specific Mortality. *Ann Int Med.* 2010 Sep;153(5):289–298.
3. Ilona Staprans; Xian-Mang Pan; Joseph H. Rapp; Kenneth R. Feingold. Oxidized Cholesterol in the Diet Accelerates the Development of Aortic Atherosclerosis in Cholesterol-Fed Rabbits *Arteriosclerosis, Thrombosis, and Vascular Biology.* 1998;18:977-983.).
4. Tappel A. Heme of consumed red meat can act as a catalyst of oxidative damage and could initiate colon, breast and prostate cancers, heart disease and other diseases. *Med Hypotheses.* 2007;68(3):562-4. Epub 2006 Oct 11.
5. Newgard, C.B. An, J. Baine, J.R., et al. A branched chain-amino acid metabolic signature that differentiates obese and lean humans and contributes to insulin resistance. *Cell Metabolism.* 2009; 9(4): 311-26.
6. Allen, N.E. et al. Life-style determinants of serum insulin-like growth factor-I (IGF-I), C-peptide and hormone binding protein levels in British Women. *Cancer Causes and Control.* .2003; 14(1): 65-74.
7. Benardot, D. Advanced Sports Nutrtition. Pg 32. Human Kinetics, 2006.
8. Stanton. R, Crowe T. Risks of a high-protein diet outweigh the benefits. *Nature.* 2006, Feb 13:440(7086:868.
9. Livestock's Long Shadow: Environmental Issues and Options. Food and Agriculture Organization of the United Nations; 2006.
10. Fuhrman, J. Do Primitive People Live Longer? From Dr Fuhrman's website:
    "Inuit Greenlanders, who historically have had limited access to fruits and vegetables, have the worst longevity statistics in North America. Research from the past and present shows that they die on an average

of about 10 years younger, and have a higher rate of cancer, than the overall Canadian population. Similar statistics are available for the high meat-consuming Maasai in Kenya. They eat a diet high in wild hunted meats, and have the worst life expectancy in the modern world. Life expectancy is 45 years for women and 42 years for men. African researchers report that historically, Maasai rarely live beyond age 60."

11. Robbins, John. *Healthy at a Hundred.* Pg 110-121. New York, NY. Balantine Books, 2006.
12. Sission, Mark, *The Primal Blueprint.* Primal Blueprint Inc. 2009. P 1-8.
13. Cordain, Loren. *The Paleo Diet.* P 40, 67, 101. New York. John Wiley and Sons. 2002.
14. Bulhões, A.C.; Goldani, H.A.S.; Oliveira, F.S.; Matte, U.S.; Mazzuca, R.B.; Silveira, T.R. Correlation between lactose absorption and the C/T-13910 and G/A-22018 mutations of the lactase-phlorizin hydrolase (LCT) gene in adult-type hypolactasia. *Brazilian Journal of Medical and Biological Research* 40 (11): 1441–6.
15. Cordain, Loren. *The Paleo Diet.* P 20-37. New York. John Wiley and Sons. 2002.
16. Eaton SB, Konner M, Paleolithic Nutrition: A consideration of its nature and current implications. *New England Journal of Medicine* 1985, Jan 31;312(5):283-9.
17. Milton, K., Hunter-gatherer diets—a different perspective. *Am J Clin Nutr* 2000 71: 665–667.
18. Milton K., Demmend M., Digestive and passage kinetics of chimpanzees fed high fiber and low fiber diets and comparison with human data. *Journal of Nutrition* 1988;118:1
19. Milton K. Hypothesis to explain the role of meat eating in human evolution. *Evolutionary Anthropology* 1999; 8:11.
20. Campbell, T. Colin. *The China Study.* P 43-68. Benbella Books, 2006.
21. Jaminet, P., Jaminnet, S.C. *Perfect Health Diet.* Yin Yang Press. 2010.
22. PerfectHealthDiet.com
23. D'Adamo, Peter. *Eat Right 4 Your Type.* New York, NY. C.P. Putman's Sons, 1996.
24. D'Adamo, Peter. *Live Right 4 Your Type.* New York, NY. C.P. Putman's Sons, 1998.

25. S. Wiener, et al. Blood groups of apes and monkeys. The ABO blood groups, secreter and Lewis types of apes. *American Journal of Physical Anthropology.* Volume 21, issue 3, pgs 271-281, Sep 1963.
26. From the South Beach Diet Website.
27. Horne, Ross. *Improving on Pritikin.* Pp 119–138. Avalon Beach, Australia. 1988.
28. Hubbard JD, Inkeles S, Barnard RJ. Nathan Pritikin's heart. N Engl J Med. 1985 Jul 4; 313(1):52.
29. Ornish, D. Can lifestyle changes reverse heart disease? *Lancet. 1990* Jul 21;*336*(8708):*129*-33.
30. Berry R. *Famous Vegetarians.*
31. Buettner, Dan. *The Blue Zone.* Washington, D.C. National Geographic Society, 2008.
32. Buettner, D. "Longevity: The Secrets of a Long Life." National Geographic Society. 2005.
33. Ehret, A. *Mucusless Diet Healing System.* Benedict Lust Publications, 2002.
34. Gerson, C., Bishop B. *Healing The Gerson Way.* Sheridan Books. 2007.
35. A. T. Hovannessian. *Raw Eating.* 3rd ed. Hallelujah Acres Publishing, Shelby NC. 2000. Originally published in 1960 by Mr. Hovannessian under the title of Raw Eating: or A New World Free From Diseases, Vices and Poisons. Mr. Hovannessian is, arguably, the "father" of the modern raw food movement. His book brought the foundational principles of the raw diet to the public eye. The roots of the modern raw food movement, including the main talking points, can be seen in his work. Apparently, this book directly or indirectly motivated and guided a number of the raw food teachers and writers in the latter 20th century. Unfortunately, some of these raw food teachers blatantly plagiarized Hovannessian's work.
36. A. T. Hovannessian. *Raw Eating.* 3rd ed. Hallelujah Acres Publishing, Shelby NC. 2000. Page 26. The author reached his conclusion after two of his children died. The first child died after conventional medical treatment. The second child was apparently recovering after adopting a raw food diet, only to regress again and eventually die after resuming a cooked food diet.
37. Steinmetz KA, et al. *Raw Vegetables and cancer.* J Am Dietary Association. 1996 (10)1027–39.

38. Barnard N.D. *Dr. Neal Barnard's Program for Reversing Diabetes*. Rodale Books, NY New York. Pp 39–57.
39. Graham, D. N. *The 80/10/10 Diet*. Pg 127. Decatur GA. FoodnSport Press, 2006.
40. Lanaspa MA, Et al. Uric Acid Induces Hepatic Steatosis by Generation of Mitochondrial Oxidative Stress: Potential toxic role in fructose dependent and independent fatty liver. *Biol Chem.* 2012 Nov 23; 287(48): 40732–44. doi: 10.1074/jbc.M112.399899.
41. Durette. R. *Fruit: The Ultimate Diet*. Fruitarian Vibes, Camp Verde, Arizona. 1999.
42. Osborne, A. *Fruitarianism, the Path to Paradise*. Queensland, Australia. 2009.
43. Fielder, J.L. (ed) *Handbook of Natural Hygiene*.

Chapter 10

1. Robbins, John. *Healthy at a Hundred*. Pg 41. New York, NY. Balantine Books, 2006.

Chapter 11

1. Those were the words of "Mr. Spock," spoken in the Star Trek movie, "The Undiscovered Country."

Chapter 12

1. Buettner, D. The Blue Zone. Pgs. 21-59. The National Geographic Society. 2008.

Chapter 13

1. Ornish D: Holy Cow! What's Good For You Is Good For Our Planet: Comment on "Red Meat Consumption and Mortality". *Arch Intern Med* 2012.
2. Selye. H. *The Stress of Life*. 1956. "Let me point out here parenthetically that Pasteur was sharply criticized for failing to recognize the importance of the terrain (the soil in which disease develops). They said

he was too one-sidedly preoccupied with the apparent cause of disease: the microbe itself. There were, in fact, many disputes about this between Pasteur and his great contemporary, Claude Bernard. The former insisted on the importance of the disease producer, the latter on the body's own equilibrium. Yet Pasteur's work on immunity induced with serums and vaccines shows he recognized the importance of the soil. In any event, it is rather significant that Pasteur attached so much importance to this point that on his deathbed he said to Professor A. Rénon who looked after him: 'Bernard avait raison. Le germe n'est rien, c'est le terrain qui est tout.' ('Bernard was right. The microbe is nothing, the soil is everything.')."

3. Hemenway, T. *Gaia's Garden.* Pg 121. Chelsea Green Publishing Company, White River Junction, Vermont. 2000..
4. Manning, R. *Against the Grain.* Northpoint Press. 2004.
5. Livestock's Long Shadow: Environmental Issues and Options. Food and Agriculture Organization of the United Nations; 2006.
6. Hemenway, T. *Gaia's Garden.* Chelsea Green Publishing Co. 2000 Pp 230–256
7. *Lettres de Marie-Antoinette*, volume I, p. 91.
8. Hemenway, T. *Gaia's Garden.* Chelsea Green Publishing Company, Wild River Junction, Vermont. 2000. P 212.
9. *Permaculture Magazine.* (From Website). 9th December 2011
10. *Permaculture Magazine.* (From Website). 3rd March 2012.
11. Tzu, Sun. *The Art of War.* p 77. Oxford University Press. 1963.
12. Tzu, Sun. *The Art of War.* p77. Oxford University Press. 1963.
13. Hemenway, T. *Gaia's Garden.* Chelsea Green Publishing Company, While River Junction, Vermont. 2000. Pp 17–18 .
14. Tzu, Sun. *The Art of War.* p 74. Oxford University Press. 1963.
15. Canticle to Brother Sun (Originally called Canticle to All Creatures) by St. Francis of Assisi.
16. The reason fasting has this effect is not entirely understood, but we do know fasting allows for a profound cleansing and physiological "resting" of the body, both of which could favor clear thinking and emotional serenity. According to one study, fasting animals show a reduction in the levels of a group of enzymes called MAO (Monoamine oxidases).[17] These enzymes help to detoxify the body. However, they also accelerate the breakdown of the brain chemicals (mono-amines)

associated with emotional calmness, joyfulness, and kindness. The reduction of these enzymes during fasting might allow for higher levels of those feel-good brain chemicals, which might account for the mental clarity and emotional serenity associated with fasting. A plant based diet might support the same process on a more subtle level by allowing the body to simply cleanse itself more easily and therefore maintain lower levels of MAO. In that regard, fruits and vegetables would be especially beneficial, for they tend to be the least toxic of the food groups, as well as containing some natural MAO inhibitors.

17. Iffiú-Soltész Z, Prévot D, Carpéné C. Influence of prolonged fasting on monoamine oxidase and semicarbazide-sensitive amine oxidase activities in rat white adipose tissue. *Journal of Physiological Biochemistry.* 2009 Mar;65(1):11–23. Source: INSERM, U858, I2MR, University Paul Sabatier of Toulouse, France.
18. Robbins, J., No Happy Cow. Canori Press. San Franscisco, CA. 2012. Pp 121–124.
19. Colbert C., Why is Haiti so Poor? The Haiti Project Newsletter. 1986.
20. Berry R., *Food for the Gods: Vegetarianism & the World's Religions.* Pythagorean Publishers. 1998
21. Tompkin, P., Bird C., *The Secret Life of Plants.* Harper Collins Publishers. 1972

Chapter 14

1. Lipton, B, H. Bhaerman, S. *Spontaneous Evolution.* Hay House. Carlsbad CA. 2009. Pp 221–242.
2. Clark, A.C. *2001, A Space Odyssey. Closing lines*: "For though he was master of the world, he was not quite sure what to do next. But he would think of something."

Appendix

1. Schatz IJ, Masaki K, Yano K, Chen R, Rodriguez BL, Curb JD. Cholesterol and all-cause mortality in elderly people from the Honolulu Heart Program: a cohort study. *Lancet.* 2001 Aug 4;358(9279):351–355.

2. Abramson J, Wright JM. Are lipid-lowering guidelines evidence-based? *Lancet.* 2007 Jan 20; 369(9557):168–9
3. Brown BG, Taylor AJ Does ENHANCE Diminish Confidence in Lowering LDL or in Ezetimibe? *Engl J Med* 358:1504, April 3, 2008 Editorial.
4. Kennel, W.B., et al. Factor of Risk in development of coronary heart disease. *Ann of Internal Medicine.* 55 (1961): 33–50.
5. Esselstyn, C.B. Updating a 12-year experience with arrest and reversal therapy for coronary eart Disease. *American Journal of Cardiology.* 84 (1999): 339–41.
6. Pencina, M.J. et al. Predicting the 30-Year Risk of Cardiovascular Disease. The Framingham Heart Study. *Circulation.* 2009; 119: 3078-3084 Published online before print June 8, 2009.
7. Esselstyn, Caldwell, B. *Prevent and Reverse Heart Disease.* 31–32. Every Books. New York. 2007.
8. Donpunha W., Kukongviriyapan U, Sompamit K, Pakongviriyan V, Pannangech P. Protective Effect of Ascorbic Acid on Cadmium-induced Hypertension and vascular Dysfunction in Mice. *Miometals.* 2011 Feb:24(1) 105–15.
9. Abeywardenia MY. Patten, GS. Role of Omega-3 long chain Polyunsaturated Fatty Acids in Reducing Cardio-Metabolic Risk Factors. *Endocr Immun Metab Disorder Drug Targets.* 2011 June 8. PMMID: 21651471.
10. Nunez-Cordoba JM, Martinez-Gonzalez MA. Antioxidant Vitamins and Cardiovascular Disease. *Curr Top Med Chem.* 2011, April 21.
11. Mora, S. LDL Particle Size: Does it Matter? M.H.S., Brigham and Women's Hospital, Harvard Medical School, Boston, Massachusetts. (article)
12. Ilona Staprans; Xian-Mang Pan; Joseph H. Rapp; Kenneth R. Feingold. Oxidized. Cholesterol in the Diet Accelerates the Development of Aortic Atherosclerosis in Cholesterol-Fed Rabbits. *Arteriosclerosis, Thrombosis, and Vascular Biology.* 1998; 18:977–983.).
13. Tappel A. Heme of consumed red meat can act as a catalyst of oxidative damage and could initiate colon, breast and prostate cancers, heart disease and other diseases. *Med Hypotheses.* 2007. 68(3):562–4. Epub 2006 Oct 11.

14. Vogel, Robert, A. Brachial Artery Ultrasound: A Noninvasive Tool in Assessment of Triglyceride Rich Lipoproteins. *Clinical Cardiology*. June 1999.
15. Holt H, Miller JC, Petocz P. Insulin Index of Foods: the insulin demand generated by 100kj portions of common foods. *Am J Cli Nutri*. 1997. 66:1264–1267.

About the Author

Rudy Scarfalloto received his Bachelor of Science degree in biology at Brooklyn College, and his Doctor of Chiropractic degree at Life Chiropractic College. He maintains a chiropractic practice in Atlanta, Georgia, specializing in low-force spinal adjusting, nutrition, and techniques for promoting the health of the internal organs. He also teaches a number of health related classes and seminars. In addition to his chiropractic practice and teaching, Dr. Scarfalloto has also published four other books: *The Dance of Opposites, Cultivating Inner Harmony, The Edge of Time,* and *Nutrition for Massage Therapists.*

Index

A
Acid and alkaline 4
Addictions 211
   Food 158
   Sugar 18
Almonds 40
Amaranth 34
Antioxidants 12
Apple juice 57
Apples 37, 57, 63
Arterial plaquing 102, 225
Atkins Diet 103
Avocados 118, 123, 124

B
B vitamins 29
Bananas 37
Barley 110
Beef 42
Beets 39
Beta Carotene 32
Blackberries 132
Blood sugar 125, 136
Blood-Type Diet 110
Broccoli 39
Bran 19, 29. 33
Brain growth and food 79
Brazil nuts 40
Bread 33
   Sprouted-grain 34
   Sourdough 34, 35
   Whole wheat 34
Blue berries 37
Buckwheat 123

Building foods 4

C
Cabbage 45
Calories 9, 10, 20, 96
Carbohydrates 15
Calcium 30
Carotenoids 31, 32
Carrot juice 51
Carrots 31, 39
Cauliflower 19
Cherries 18
Cholesterol 21
Celery 39
Cleansing foods 4
Coconuts 123
Coconut milk 46
Complex carbohydrates 18
Corn 33
Cucumbers 38

D
DHA 24, 26
Dandelion 39
Dairy 42, 43
Digestion 56

E
Eggs 42, 43
Emotions 58, 141
Emotional eating 145
Enzymes 12
EPA 24, 26
Ethics of eating 181

F
Fats 20
Fermented foods 44
Fiber 18
Figs 38
Fish 41
Fitness and food 178
Flavonoids 31, 32
Flax seeds 40
Food as medicine 10-11
Food Combining 62-63
Fructose 17
Fruit 38
   As a staple food 134
   High fruit diet 124
   100% fruit diet 129
Fruit juice 18, 57, 59
Fuhrman's Diet 117

G
Galactose 16
Grains 32
Grapes 38
Glucose 38, 39
Gluten-free Diet 110

H
Homocysteine 114, 126, 176
Hominids 78
Hormones 12

I
Iodine 31
Instincts 55, 98, 99
Instinctual eating 151, 160-162
Iron 30

J
Juicing 145

K
Kale 39
Kidneys 40, 52, 53, 57, 104
Kiwi fruit 38, 136, 141

L
Lactose 17, 43, 44
Large Intestine 56
Legumes 36
Lentils 36, 45, 54
Liver 39, 57
Low-carb diets 10-102, 118
Low-fat diets 113, 118
Lungs 58

M
Macrobiotic Diet 44, 114, 137
Macronutrients 8-10, 30
Magnesium 30
Mangos 132
Micronutrients 8-10, 114
Milk 42-43
Millet 33, 110
Minerals 30, 33, 36, 38
Miso 35, 44
Monosaccharides 16
Monounsaturated fats 21

N
Natto 35, 36
Natural Hygiene 133
Neanderthal 83-84
Neolithic Period 85
Nutrients 6
Nuts 4, 24, 39
Nut and seed milk 47

O
Oats 33
Oils 20
Olive oil 23
Olives 143, 163
Omega-3 24
Omega-6 24
Orange juice 58, 135
Organically grown food 65
Ornish Diet 115
Oxidized oils 26

P

Paleolithic Diet 71, 106-107, 137
Paleolithic Period 83-84, 88, 106, 107
Partially hydrogenated oils 25
Papaya 38
Peanuts 35
Permaculture 189, 194, 197, 216
Phytonutrients 28
Pineapple 38
Polysaccharides 16
Polyunsaturated 22
Pomegranates 38
Potassium 30
Price, Weston A. 104, 106
Primal Diet 106
Primates 88, 127, 163, 216-217
Primate diet 73, 91, 127
Pritikin Diet 115
Protein 27
   Requirements 27
   Toxicity 52
Poultry 43
Prunes 38
Pumpkin seeds 40

Q

Quinoa 32

R

Raw food diets 120
Rice 32

S

Saturated fats 21-22
Sauerkraut 44
Selenium 30
Sesame seeds 40
Slavery and grain farming 212
Sodium 30
South Beach Diet 112
Soy 35-36
Spinach 39
Starch 18

Steroids 20
Strawberries 39
Sucrose 17
Sugars 16
   Natural 17
   Refined 17
Sulfur 31, 39, 102, 121
Sunflower seeds 40

T

Tempeh 44
Thoreau, Henry David 152, 213
Tofu 36
Tomatoes 38
Toxins 10, 49
Triglycerides 21

U

Unsaturated fats 21-22

V

Vegetable juice 123, 131
Vegetarian Diet 117
Vegan Diet 117
Vitamin A 29, 87
Vitamin B1 29
Vitamin B3 29
Vitamin B5 29
Vitamin B12 29, 30
Vitamin C 29, 30, 87
Vitamin D 29
Vitamin E 29
Vitamin K 29

W

Walnuts 40
Water 12-13
Watermelon 38, 57
Weight loss 101, 108, 117
Weston A. Price Diet 104, 105
Weston A. Price Foundation 105
Whole food 7-8

Z
Zinc 31
Zone Diet 109
Zucchini 129-130

Made in the USA
Charleston, SC
01 June 2014